A Handbook for

Student Nurses

Third edition

3rd edition

2019-20

Lantern

A Handbook for

Student Nurses

Introducing Key Issues Relevant for Practice

Wendy Benbow, Gill Jordan, Anneyce Knight and Sara White

2267

KH

ISBN 9781908625755

First edition published in 2009 by Reflect Press Ltd (ISBN 9781906052195)

Second edition published in 2013 by Lantern Publishing Ltd (ISBN 9781908625144)

2015–16 edition published in 2015 by Lantern Publishing Ltd (ISBN 9781908625359)

2016–17 edition published in 2015 by Lantern Publishing Ltd (ISBN 9781908625373)

2017–18 edition published in 2017 by Lantern Publishing Ltd (ISBN 9781908625434)

2018–19 edition published in 2018 by Lantern Publishing Ltd (ISBN 9781908625571)

Third edition published in 2019

Lantern Publishing Limited, The Old Hayloft, Vantage Business Park, Bloxham Rd, Banbury, OX16 9UX, UK

www.lanternpublishing.com

British Library Cataloguing in Publication Data

A catalogue record for this book is available from the British Library

The authors and publisher have made every attempt to ensure the content of this book is up to date and accurate. However, healthcare knowledge and information is changing all the time so the reader is advised to double-check any information in this text on drug usage, treatment procedures, the use of equipment, etc. to confirm that it complies with the latest safety recommendations, standards of practice and legislation, as well as local Trust policies and procedures. Students are advised to check with their tutor and/or practice supervisor before carrying out any of the procedures in this textbook.

Typeset by Medlar Publishing Solutions Pvt Ltd, India
Cover design by Andrew Magee Design Ltd.
Printed in the UK
Last digit is the print number: 10 9 8 7 6 5 4 3

CONTENTS

PREFACE TO THE THIRD EDITION

The Nursing and Midwifery Council (NMC) is the regulatory body for nurses and midwives and is responsible for setting standards of proficiency. The standards of proficiency define the overarching principles of being able to practise as a nurse, and must be achieved before students are eligible to join the register. The aim of this handbook is to highlight and address many of the key issues which surround these standards of proficiency and relate them to not only the working knowledge you require in the practice setting but also to *The Code: professional standards of practice and behaviour for nurses, midwives and nursing associates.*

This handbook has been written for student nurses, return to practice nurses and those who trained overseas, students undertaking Further Education Access courses or BTEC (Business and Technology Education Council) qualifications, and Nursing Associates. The content is also relevant for healthcare assistants and assistant practitioners, as many of the principles are relevant to all those working in care settings. It is designed so that each individual chapter can be utilised as a quick source of reference, although together with the activities and further reading, it may serve as a starting point for more in-depth study.

Anneyce Knight and Sara White
May 2019

ACTIVITIES AND QR CODES

In some of the Activities in this book we have used QR codes to enable you to reach websites quickly and easily. Download a QR reader/scanner onto your smartphone, scan the code and it will take you instantly to the relevant website.

PREFACE TO THE SECOND EDITION

The NMC is responsible for setting standards of proficiency that define the overarching principles of being able to practise as a nurse, and must be achieved before students are eligible to join the register. The aim of this handbook is to highlight and address many of the key issues which surround these standards of proficiency and relate them to working knowledge you require in the practice setting.

The handbook has been written primarily for student nurses, return to practice nurses and those who trained overseas, but it is envisaged that students undertaking Further Education access courses and Qualifications and Credit Framework (QCF) courses in health care will also find the information helpful. The content is also relevant for Health Care Assistants and Assistant Practitioners.

The information within the book is relevant to all areas of nursing, and all branches of nursing. It is designed so that you can utilise individual chapters as a quick source of reference, although along with the activities and further reading, it may serve as a starting point for more in-depth study. Where websites are identified, these are only suggested sources of further information and others may be found through general search engines such as www.google.co.uk. Although the emphasis is mainly related to healthcare in England, we do refer to Scotland, Wales and Northern Ireland when appropriate.

Wendy Benbow and Gill Jordan

ABOUT THE AUTHORS

Wendy Benbow: Following qualification as a registered nurse in 1969, Wendy worked for two years in genito-urinary surgery and major spinal injuries before moving into community nursing. Over a fourteen-year period Wendy was involved in a variety of roles that included community nursing sister, practice work teacher and nurse manager, as well as time seconded for research and coordinating pre-registration student placements for the local acute hospital. After a year out to complete her teaching qualification, Wendy began working full-time in education in 1985. She was involved in both teaching on and managing a range of pre- and post-registration courses, programme development, regionally funded research and national project development. Wendy has now retired from working in healthcare.

Gill Jordan: On qualifying as a registered nurse in 1978, Gill completed her Orthopaedic Nursing Certificate and moved to New Zealand where she worked in a large orthopaedic teaching hospital, ultimately as a ward sister of a trauma orthopaedic ward. On her return to the UK in 1988, Gill moved into nurse education. Since then, she has been involved in a variety of courses and professional development programmes, as both a teacher and programme leader. These have included courses leading to professional registration, Return to Practice, Overseas Nurses Programme, conversion courses and various post-registration undergraduate and postgraduate programmes. Gill has now retired from working in healthcare.

Anneyce Knight: Anneyce is currently a Senior Lecturer in Adult Nursing at Bournemouth University and Programme Leader for the Return to Practice (Nursing) course. She qualified as a registered nurse in 1982 and worked in orthopaedics and oncology, then trained as a midwife. She continued to practise in a variety of nursing and midwifery clinical settings before moving into Higher Education in 2000. Prior to taking up her current role in 2015, Anneyce was the Course Lead for the innovative Foundation Degree in Health and Social Care (clinical) for Associate Practitioners, a joint NHS and Southampton Solent University collaboration. Previously she was at the University of Greenwich, where she held a number of positions. She is passionate about the need for compassionate care, thereby enhancing the quality of patient care, particularly at the end of life. Her primary research interests focus on Public Health and Wellbeing, areas in which she has published and presented nationally and internationally.

Sara White: Sara qualified as a registered nurse in 1986, after which she worked in Acute Trauma and Orthopaedics before moving to Intensive care (ICU) and Coronary care. She worked in a number of ICUs in London and the south of England and gained multiple qualifications (including General Intensive Care Nursing, Principles of Intensive Care (Paediatrics), BSc (Hons) Nursing Studies and Diploma in Health Service Management). Having spent ten years as an ICU Sister she moved into Higher Education (HEI) where she has been for twenty years. During her time in HEI she has facilitated the learning of many thousands of students at both undergraduate level and postgraduate level, whilst at the same time continuing her own education to Doctorate level. She believes that as a nurse educator she should strive to enable students to fuse their learning and integrate education, professional practice and research in order to develop as future nurses and enhance the care they offer patients.

NURSE EDUCATION, PRACTICE SUPERVISION AND ASSESSMENT

This chapter provides an overview of the current context of nursing and the preparation nurses undertake during their pre-registration programmes, and an insight into the registered nurse's role in supporting students.

LEARNING OUTCOMES

On completion of this chapter you should:
- have an awareness of the needs of the 21st century nurse, and of programmes leading to nurse registration
- have an understanding of *Future Nurse*, the regulatory body's standards of proficiency for registered nurses (NMC, 2018a)
- understand the role of practice supervisors and assessors in nursing
- be able to define the qualities required to be a good practice supervisor and assessor

>> Introduction

First things first – welcome to your nursing course! This is the start of your journey to becoming a qualified, registered nurse with a university degree, confident and competent to provide compassionate care to all your patients and service users.

In this chapter we will look at the sort of education and training you can expect, and the standards you will be expected to meet. In addition to achieving the proficiencies established by the Nursing and Midwifery Council (NMC), which is the regulatory body overseeing the profession, you must also remember that as a nursing student and when you are a registered nurse you are a role model for your profession and you are required to adhere to the NMC's (2018e) *The Code: professional standards of practice and behaviour for nurses, midwives and nursing associates* (hereafter abbreviated to the *Code*).

We wish you success in your studies and in your career as a registered nurse. And now down to business.

>> Pre-registration nurse education

Background

At the end of your nurse education you will leave with not only a first-level professional nursing qualification (registered nurse), but also a university degree. This was not always the case and today there are many different routes to gaining nurse registration, such as nurse apprentice, BSc (Hons) Nursing, BA (Hons) Nursing, postgraduate diploma, Master's and combined courses such as BSc (Hons) Nursing and Midwifery or BSc (Hons) Adult and Mental Health Nursing. These programmes vary from between two and four years full time, and up to five or six years part time. However, whichever route you take, at entry point to the NMC register, standards need to be met.

Nurse education in the UK has undergone many changes over the last few decades, as nurses embrace the many rapid changes in society. These include an ever-increasing

>> Nursing is a profession for the intellectually curious, lifelong learner.

range of healthcare responsibilities, an ageing population and growing rates of diabetes, obesity and other conditions. This means the healthcare system is dealing with an increasing number of complex illnesses, and increasing pressure on staffing and budgets.

It is difficult to give a comprehensive picture of these changes, but an influential report was produced by Lord Willis in March 2015 (Health Education England, 2015) in which he made recommendations for nurse education. These included a clear pathway and distinct qualifications for care assistants and a change to the structure of pre-registration education. He proposed that greater acquisition of skills which were previously considered 'advanced' or post-registration be included within pre-registration education, and that the emphasis of a pre-registration programme should be on developing greater decision-making skills and the involvement of patients in shared decision-making and the routine application of research and innovation.

Today's nurses are not just caring for the sick, they are very much involved in the notion of modern medicine and healthcare delivery: they give talks, actively address healthcare policy, publish research, develop mobile medical applications (medical apps) and collaborate with other healthcare colleagues, administrators and nurse educators. Nursing has become more complex, in ways that could not have been imagined a generation or two ago. The demands of healthcare are calling for a new generation of thinkers who want to be agents of care innovation. Nursing therefore is a profession for the intellectually curious, lifelong learner. Nevertheless, there need to be standards in nurse education.

» Nurse education today

The NMC sets the standards for pre-registration nursing education (Nursing and Midwifery (Amendment) Order, 2016). These are articulated in *Future Nurse: standards of proficiency for registered nurses* (NMC, 2018a). When using the standards, it is important also to read *Realising Professionalism: standards for education and training*, which consists of three parts:

- *Part 1: Standards framework for nursing and midwifery education* (NMC, 2018b)
- *Part 2: Standards for student supervision and assessment* (NMC, 2018c) and
- *Part 3: Standards for pre-registration nursing programmes* (NMC, 2018d).

These documents provide a complete picture of what nurses need to know and be able to do, by the time they register with the NMC; they also detail what approved education institutions and their practice placement partners must provide. There are separate standards for midwives.

The Royal College of Nursing (RCN, 2014, p. 3) states that the defining characteristics of nursing are:

> » A professional person achieving a competent standard of practice following successful completion of an approved education programme will be a nurse who is a safe, caring and competent decision-maker.

1. A particular **purpose**: the purpose of nursing is to promote health, healing, growth and development, and to prevent disease, illness, injury and disability. When people become ill or disabled, the purpose of nursing is, in addition, to minimise distress and suffering, and to enable people to understand and cope with their disease or disability, its treatment and its consequences. When death is inevitable, the purpose of nursing is to maintain the best possible quality of life until its end.
2. A particular **mode of intervention**: nursing interventions are concerned with empowering people, and helping them to achieve, maintain or recover independence. Nursing is an intellectual, physical, emotional and moral process which includes the identification of nursing needs; therapeutic interventions and personal care; information, education, advice and advocacy; and physical, emotional and spiritual support. In addition to direct patient care, nursing practice includes management, teaching, and policy and knowledge development.
3. A particular **domain**: the specific domain of nursing is people's unique responses to and experience of health, illness, frailty, disability and health-related life events in whatever environment or circumstances they find themselves. People's responses may be physiological, psychological, social, cultural or spiritual, and are often a combination of all of these.

The term 'people' includes individuals of all ages, families and communities, throughout the entire lifespan.

4. *A particular focus: the focus of nursing is the whole person and the human response rather than a particular aspect of the person or a particular pathological condition.*

5. *A particular value base: nursing is based on ethical values which respect the dignity, autonomy and uniqueness of human beings, the privileged nurse–patient relationship and the acceptance of personal accountability for decisions and actions. These values are expressed in written codes of ethics, and supported by a system of professional regulation.*

6. *A commitment to partnership: nurses work in partnership with patients, their relatives and other carers, and in collaboration with others as members of a multidisciplinary team. Where appropriate, they will lead the team, prescribing, delegating and supervising the work of others; at other times they will participate under the leadership of others. At all times, however, they remain personally and professionally accountable for their own decisions and actions.*

Consequently, a professional person achieving a competent standard of practice following successful completion of an approved education programme will be a nurse who is a safe, caring and competent decision-maker. A nurse is also willing to accept personal and professional accountability for their actions and continuous learning. The nurse practises within a statutory framework and code of ethics delivering nursing practice (care) that is appropriately based on research, evidence and critical thinking that effectively responds to the needs of individual clients (patients) and diverse populations.

The NMC does not produce a national curriculum for nursing education, but it does determine the content of programmes. Equally, the NMC does not set specific requirements for the nature or range of practice learning, other than that it must enable the competencies to be acquired. University programmes have to be validated by the NMC, and are subject to regular reviews. In addition to NMC standards, universities also have to comply with standards set by the Quality Assurance Agency (QAA), which are general standards for all courses run within higher education.

Normally students enrol on a programme of one or two (for joint programmes) of the four fields of nursing practice (adult, children, learning disabilities, mental health). Whichever field is studied, 50 per cent of time is spent on theoretical aspects of nursing and 50 per cent either in simulation or in practice areas. This equates to 2300 hours each of practice and theory (4600 hours in total) with progression points at the end of each year, where both theory and practice competencies have to be achieved.

» Standards of proficiency for registered nurses

The NMC has to be satisfied that its standards for granting a person a licence to practise are being met as required, and it does this by setting proficiencies and competencies that must be achieved before you are eligible to join the register. As discussed, these standards are set out in the NMC document *Future Nurse: standards of proficiency for registered nurses* (NMC, 2018a), which replaced the previous 2014 *Standards for Competence for Registered Nurses* (NMC, 2014) following a long period of consultation. Professional standards are very important, because nurses are expected to:

- uphold professional values
- have effective communication and interpersonal skills
- be effective decision-makers
- have management, leadership and teamworking skills.

Together with standards, the ability to deliver essential skills is also very important; these skills are shown below in *Annexe A*.

The NMC standards of proficiency, and nursing practice in general, have been informed by other documents in addition to the Willis Report (Health Education England, 2015):

- In 2012 Cummings and Bennett, writing for the Department of Health, authored *Compassion in Practice: nursing, midwifery and care staff – our vision and strategy.* This included the '6Cs' – Care, Compassion, Courage, Communication, Competence and Commitment, which were referred to as 'our fundamental values' (see also *Chapter 3*).
- This was followed up by NHS England publishing *Leading Change, Adding Value* (NHS England, 2016). This publication built upon *Compassion in Practice* and underpins the NHS *Five Year Forward View* (NHS, 2016) plan.
- This *Five Year Forward View* (NHS, 2016) plan focused on seeking to develop new ways of working which are person-centred and which provide seamless care across the boundary that has traditionally separated health and social care. The plan identified three crucial gaps in the NHS: health and wellbeing; care and quality; and funding and efficiency (see also *Chapter 8*).

ACTIVITY 1.1

Access *Compassion in Practice* using the link below or by scanning the QR code, and review the 6Cs. What do they mean to you? How can you ensure you uphold these in practice?

www.england.nhs.uk/wp-content/uploads/2012/12/compassion-in-practice.pdf

Within the standards of proficiency for registered nurses (NMC, 2018a) there are seven platforms:
1. Being an accountable professional
2. Promoting health and preventing ill health
3. Assessing needs and planning care
4. Providing and evaluating care
5. Leading and managing nursing care and working in teams
6. Improving safety and quality of care
7. Coordinating care.

The NMC (2018a) states that "The outcome statements for each platform have been designed to apply across all four fields of nursing practice (adult, children, learning disabilities, mental health) and all care settings". When these have been achieved, the NMC feels that the public can be confident that all new nurses will:
- represent the knowledge, skills and attributes that all registered nurses must demonstrate when caring for people of all ages and across all care settings
- reflect what the public can expect nurses to know and be able to do in order to deliver safe, compassionate and effective nursing care
- provide a benchmark for nurses from the European Economic Area (EEA), the European Union (EU) and overseas wishing to join the register
- provide a benchmark for those who plan to return to practice after a period of absence.

There are two annexes to the NMC (2018a) standards of proficiency which provide a description of what registered nurses should be able to demonstrate they can do at the point of registration in order to provide safe nursing care. *Annexe A* specifies the communication and relationship management skills required, and *Annexe B* specifies the nursing procedures that registered nurses must demonstrate that they are able to perform safely. As with the knowledge proficiencies, the annexes also identify where more advanced skills are required by registered nurses, working in a particular field of nursing practice.

Annexe A: Communication and relationship management skills

The skills outlined in this annexe, which all registered nurses must demonstrate with all patients and their families and carers, are set out in four sections:
1. Underpinning communication skills for assessing, planning, providing and managing best practice, evidence-based nursing care.
2. Evidence-based, best practice approaches to communication for supporting people of all ages, their families and carers in preventing ill health and in managing their care.

3. Evidence-based, best practice communication skills and approaches for providing therapeutic interventions.
4. Evidence-based, best practice communication skills and approaches for working with people in professional teams.

After each of these statements there are between nine and fifteen areas that must be met. For example, the registered nurse should:

- actively listen, recognise and respond to verbal and non-verbal cues
- use prompts and positive verbal and non-verbal reinforcement
- share information and check understanding about the causes, implications and treatment of a range of common health conditions including anxiety, depression, memory loss, diabetes, dementia, respiratory disease, cardiac disease, neurological disease, cancer, skin problems, immune deficiencies, psychosis, stroke and arthritis
- make use of motivational interviewing techniques, solution-focused therapies and reminiscence therapies
- demonstrate effective supervision, teaching and performance appraisal through the use of clear instructions and explanations when supervising, teaching or appraising others
- demonstrate effective person and team management.

ACTIVITY 1.2

You may already have some of the communication skills outlined in the NMC document. Download the standards of proficiency from the NMC website at www.nmc.org.uk/standards/standards-for-nurses/ (also available via the QR code on the right), read through Annexe A and make a note of those skills that you feel you will need to focus on first in your communication skills module.

Annexe B: Nursing procedures

In this annexe the NMC states how the registered nurse must be able not only to undertake procedures effectively but also to provide compassionate, evidence-based person-centred nursing care. This holistic approach to the care of people is essential; indeed all nursing procedures

>> The registered nurse must be able to undertake nursing procedures and also provide compassionate care.

and care should be carried out in a way which reflects cultural awareness and ensures that the needs, priorities, expertise and preferences of people are always valued and taken into account.

Annexe B Part 1 discusses the necessary procedures for assessing people's needs for person-centred care. *Part 2* discusses the procedures for the planning, provision and management of person-centred nursing care and the use of evidence-based, best practice approaches for meeting needs for care and support with rest, sleep, comfort and the maintenance of dignity, accurately assessing the person's capacity for independence and self-care and initiating appropriate interventions.

RECAP

- The Nursing and Midwifery Council (NMC) regulates the profession and sets the standards that registered nurses must meet.
- These standards are set out in the NMC document *Future Nurse: standards of proficiency for registered nurses.*
- On successful completion of your nursing course, you will have a university degree in addition to your professional qualification.

» Standards for education

You have read how the NMC expects student nurses and registered nurses to meet the required standards of proficiency and uphold the *Code*; higher education establishments are also expected to uphold standards for the education of student nurses. The NMC document *Standards framework for nursing and midwifery education* (2018b, p. 6), which is Part 1 of *Realising Professionalism: standards for education and training*, suggests that the theoretical components of the undergraduate nurse education programme include a learning culture that prioritises the safety of people, including carers, students and educators, and enables the values of the *Code* to be upheld, whilst the education and training is valued in all learning environments.

Your education institution must be approved by the NMC, and that institution, together with its practice learning partners, must:

1.1 *demonstrate that the safety of people is a primary consideration in all learning environments*

1.2 *prioritise the wellbeing of people promoting critical self-reflection and safe practice in accordance with The Code* [NMC, 2018e]

1.3 *ensure people have the opportunity to give and if required, withdraw, their informed consent to students being involved in their care*

1.4 *ensure educators and others involved in supervision, learning and assessment understand their role in preserving public safety*

1.5 ensure students and educators understand how to raise concerns or complaints and are encouraged and supported to do so in line with local and national policies without fear of adverse consequences

1.6 ensure any concerns or complaints are investigated and dealt with effectively

1.7 ensure concerns or complaints affecting the wellbeing of people are addressed immediately and effectively

1.8 ensure mistakes and incidents are fully investigated and learning reflections and actions are recorded and disseminated

1.9 ensure students are supported and supervised in being open and honest with people in accordance with the professional duty of candour

1.10 ensure the learning culture is fair, impartial, transparent, fosters good relations between individuals and diverse groups, and is compliant with equalities and human rights legislation

1.11 promote programme improvement and advance equality of opportunity through effective use of information and data

1.12 ensure programmes are designed, developed, delivered, evaluated and co-produced with service users and other stakeholders

1.13 work with service providers to demonstrate and promote inter-professional learning and working, and

1.14 support opportunities for research collaboration and evidence-based improvement in education and service provision.

Section 3 of this document is headed *Student empowerment* and speaks about how students "must be provided with a variety of learning opportunities and appropriate resources which enable them to achieve proficiencies and programme outcomes and be capable of demonstrating the professional behaviours in *The Code*" (NMC, 2018e). They note how students should be "empowered and supported to become resilient, caring, reflective and lifelong learners who are capable of working in inter-professional and inter-agency teams" (NMC 2018b, p. 9).

>> Practice placements

Nursing is both an academic discipline and a practice-based profession, so practice placements will form an essential part of your learning. They are designed to give you practical experience under supervision in a professional setting and also to enable you to demonstrate your skills and knowledge and to be assessed.

Part 2 of *Realising Professionalism: standards for education and training* discusses standards for student supervision and assessment. It describes the principles of student supervision in the practice environment and the role of practice supervisors and practice assessors. Practice learning and assessment are an essential and integral part of a nurse education programme and students are facilitated effectively and objectively by appropriately qualified and experienced professionals who have the necessary expertise for their roles.

Many practice-based professions, including nursing, traditionally rely on clinical staff to support, supervise and teach students in practice settings – the underlying rationale being that in working alongside practitioners, students will learn from experts in a safe, supportive and educationally adjusted environment (Benner, 1984). Consequently, within nursing the terms 'practice supervisor' and 'practice assessor' are generally used to describe a person who supports and assesses student nurses, while the term 'preceptor' is used for a supporter of a post-registration nurse during their first few months after qualifying (see also *Chapter 9*). You are also likely to hear the term 'mentor' in practice as this has been a term used for many years and prior to the publication of the new NMC standards in 2018.

Practice supervisors

When in practice you will be assigned to a practice supervisor. Practice supervisors must be registered with a professional regulator (such as the NMC, Health and Care Professions Council (HCPC) or General Medical Council (GMC)) and therefore you may be supervised by a nurse, a physiotherapist, a radiographer, pharmacist, occupational therapist or similar, who will help you learn. The practice supervisor is expected to:

- serve as a role model for safe and effective practice in line with their code of conduct
- support learning in line with their scope of practice to enable the student to meet their proficiencies
- support and supervise students, providing feedback on their progress towards, and achievement of, proficiencies and skills
- have current knowledge and experience of the area in which they are providing support, supervision and feedback
- contribute to the student's record of achievement by periodically recording relevant observations on the conduct, proficiency and achievement of the students they are supervising
- contribute to student assessments to inform decisions for progression
- have sufficient opportunities to engage with practice assessors and academic assessors to share relevant observations on the conduct, proficiency and achievement of the students they are supervising, and
- appropriately raise and respond to student conduct and competence concerns and be supported in doing so.

(NMC, 2018c)

In order for registered healthcare professionals to be effective supervisors, the NMC expects higher education establishments and practice partners to "receive ongoing support to prepare, reflect and develop for effective supervision and contribution to, student learning and assessment, and have understanding of the proficiencies and programme outcomes they are supporting students to achieve" (NMC 2018c, p. 8).

The Royal College of Nursing commissioned a Mentorship Project in 2015 entitled *From Today's Support in Practice to Tomorrow's Vision for Excellence* (RCN, 2016) and this project found five overarching themes that emerged following analysis of the data. These are:
1. the importance of good mentorship
2. investment in mentorship and mentors
3. relationships to enable and support mentorship
4. the context within which mentorship occurs
5. different approaches to mentorship.

This study confirms that students need a well-educated practice supervisor who is supported by the employing organisation with time and resources. Consequently, as highlighted above, practice supervisors are expected to have the skills to enable you to undergo appropriate and valuable learning experiences. They have often been qualified for a year or more and have undergone appropriate education about the role and the expectations. This may include:
• establishing effective working relationships
• facilitation of learning
• assessment and accountability
• evaluation of learning
• creating an environment for learning
• context of practice
• evidence-based practice
• leadership.

As you can see there is an expectation and requirement that all registered nurses and other healthcare practitioners play a key part in the preparation of students for registration. This is emphasised explicitly in the *Code* (NMC, 2018e, Clause 9.4), which states that registered nurses must "support students' ... learning to help them develop their professional competence and confidence" and in Part 2 of *Realising Professionalism* (NMC, 2018c).

ACTIVITY 1.3

Take a few minutes to answer the following questions:
- What qualities would you like to see in your practice supervisor?
- Can you think of any obstacles to being an effective practice supervisor?
- What are the benefits to you as a student of having a practice supervisor?

Practice supervisors are there to offer you support and guidance, and to help you make sense of your practice through:
- the application of theory
- assessing, evaluating and giving constructive feedback
- facilitating reflection on practice, performance and experiences.

Supervisors are required to comply with all standards and requirements in Part 1 of the NMC's *Realising Professionalism: standards for education and training* (NMC 2018b, p. 12) and:
- act as professional role models at all times
- receive relevant induction, ongoing support and access to education and training which includes training in equality and diversity
- have supported time and resources to enable them to fulfil their roles in addition to their other professional responsibilities
- respond effectively to the learning needs of individuals
- be supportive and objective in their approach to student supervision and assessment
- liaise and collaborate with colleagues and partner organisations in their approach to supervision and assessment
- are expected to respond effectively to concerns and complaints about public protection and student performance in learning environments, and are supported in doing so
- receive and act upon constructive feedback from students and the people they engage with to enhance the effectiveness of their teaching, supervision and assessment
- share effective practice and learn from others
- appropriately share and use evidence to make decisions on student assessment and progression.

Therefore, practice placements provide unique learning experiences and opportunities for you as a student, and the higher education provider and the practice partner ensure that these are planned, structured, managed and coordinated in order to enable you to develop professional competencies that cannot be readily acquired elsewhere. During your practice placement opportunities and practice hours you are deemed supernumerary, which means that you are not included in the permanent staff numbers. However, you are generally expected to complete the same shift patterns as your practice supervisor, and to gain experience of night working.

The NMC, in reflecting European Union requirements (Keighley, 2009), stipulates that your practice experience must include direct contact with healthy and/or sick individuals, and it must enable you to meet all your relevant statutory requirements. All your hours must be verified. The nature of your placements has to be extensive in order to provide learning opportunities that reflect the large range of healthcare needs experienced by the population, but the timing, length and type of placement will differ between individual universities.

Practice assessors

As stated above, one of the major roles of the practice supervisor is to supervise you in practice. The practice assessor's role is to assess you on your practice. Assessments and confirmation of proficiencies are based on an understanding of the student's achievements. The NMC (2018c, Section 7, p. 10) states that practice assessors must:

- conduct assessments to confirm student achievement of proficiencies
- make assessment decisions informed by feedback sought and received from practice supervisors
- make and record objective, evidence-based assessments on conduct, proficiency and achievement, drawing on student records, direct observations, student self-reflection and other resources
- maintain current knowledge and expertise relevant for the proficiencies and programme outcomes they are assessing
- work in partnership with the nominated academic assessor to evaluate and recommend the student for progression for each part of the programme, in line with programme standards and local and national policies.

As can be seen, your consistency of performance is measured via continuous assessment which is, for the most part, by your practice supervisor and/or assessor directly observing the care that you deliver.

Your own responsibilities

However, it is not only your practice supervisors and assessors who have responsibilities to you; you also have a responsibility (RCN, 2016) to:

- be proactive in seeking out experiences for your level of practice and competence with the support of your practice assessor
- demonstrate a willingness to work as part of the team in the delivery of safe patient care

- learn to express your needs and adopt a questioning, reflective approach to your learning within the multidisciplinary team
- use your practice assessor for guidance and support to enable you to achieve your learning outcomes and satisfactorily complete your practice assessments
- seek help from appropriate clinical managers or link lecturers if the practice assessor relationship is not working, to enable the achievement of the learning outcomes
- ensure that clinical skills required at each stage in the programme are attempted under the supervision of a skilled practitioner, with comments provided by both you and your practice assessor
- utilise learning opportunities outside the practice placements and, where possible, work with specialist practitioners
- identify the role of professionals within other contexts of the organisation or community; for example, in X-ray, pharmacy and outpatients
- give and receive constructive feedback
- reflect on your progress to increase self-awareness, confidence and competence.

You must also (RCN, 2016):
- read the charter and student handbooks of your higher education institution (HEI)
- familiarise yourself with handbooks related to your specific programme (these will include assessment of practice documentation)
- recognise the purpose of your placement experience and ensure you are clear about the expectations of the placement provider
- ensure you have some theoretical knowledge relating to the placement
- contact your placement and practice assessor prior to starting
- highlight any support needs to your practice assessor
- act professionally with regard to punctuality, attitude and image, and dress according to uniform policy
- maintain confidentiality
- maintain effective communication with patients, practice assessors and link personnel from both the placement and HEI.

The RCN (2017) developed a toolkit called *Helping Students Get the Best From Their Practice Placements*. The RCN speaks of the importance of effective practice-based learning, the responsibilities of stakeholders and getting the best from your practice-based learning.

This toolkit is designed to enable you, as a student of nursing or midwifery, to:
- recognise and value quality placement experiences as vital for your effective education
- optimise the support of mentors, co- and associate mentors, and others who will support your learning

- take personal responsibility for directing your own learning, making the best use of available resources
- recognise opportunities for achieving competencies for entry to the professional register
- act on the opportunity to provide honest, evaluative feedback of your practice experiences to aid the audit process for the practice placement that in turn will influence the quality of the practice placements at a local level.

ACTIVITY 1.4

Download a copy of this document and read through it:

www.rcn.org.uk/professional-development/publications/pub-006035

FURTHER READING

Clinical Placements, a book published in 2017 in Lantern Publishing's *Pocket Guides for Student Nurses* series, was written by two students, Kirstie Paterson and Jessica Wallar, to help other students make the most of their practice placements.

Academic assessors

Your educational establishment will assign you an academic assessor; these may be called a personal tutor, an academic advisor or similar, and part of their role is to "collate and confirm student achievement of proficiencies and programme outcomes in the academic environment for each part of the programme" (NMC 2018c, part 9, p. 12). Academic assessors are expected to:

- make and record objective, evidence-based decisions on conduct, proficiency and achievement, and recommendations for progression, drawing on student records and other resources
- work in partnership with a nominated practice assessor to evaluate and recommend the student for progression for each part of the programme, in line with programme standards and local and national policies
- have an understanding of the student's learning and achievement in practice.

So as you can see, when on a nurse education programme your achievements are supported and assessed by practice and education staff. They want you to achieve and become a registered nurse.

>> Registration

The title 'registered nurse' is protected in law and can only be used by someone registered with the NMC. On successful completion of your course, your university will send your course and personal details to the NMC. Your course/programme leader or director will also complete a declaration of good health and good character on your behalf, which must be received by the NMC before you can apply to register. When they have the necessary information from your university you will receive details from the NMC of how to apply for entry to the register.

Once registered, you are accountable to the NMC and have to abide by its standards and guidelines, most importantly the *Code* (NMC, 2018e) – and you will be a qualified nurse.

CHAPTER SUMMARY

- The NMC sets the standards for pre-registration.
- All courses leading to registration are 50 per cent practice and 50 per cent theory.
- All students have to achieve NMC practice proficiencies to enable them to register, and are allocated a practice assessor who assesses them in their clinical placements.

References

Benner, P. (1984) *From Novice to Expert.* California: Addison-Wesley.

Cummings, J. and Bennett, V. for the Department of Health (2012) *Compassion in Practice: nursing, midwifery and care staff – our vision and strategy.* Available at: www.england.nhs.uk/wp-content/uploads/2012/12/compassion-in-practice.pdf (accessed 3 April 2019)

Health Education England (2015) *Shape of Caring: a review of the future education and training of registered nurses and care assistants.* London: Health Education England.

Keighley, T. (2009) *The European Union Standards for Nursing and Midwifery: information for accession countries,* 2nd edition. Copenhagen, Denmark: WHO Region Office for Europe. Available at: http://apps.who.int/iris/handle/10665/107957 (accessed 3 April 2019)

NHS (2016) *Five Year Forward View.* Available at: www.england.nhs.uk/wp-content/uploads/2014/10/5yfv-web.pdf (accessed 3 April 2019)

NHS England (2016) *Leading Change, Adding Value.* Available at: www.england.nhs.uk/wp-content/uploads/2016/05/nursing-framework.pdf (accessed 3 April 2019)

Nursing and Midwifery (amendment) Order (2016). Available at: www.gov.uk/government/uploads/system/uploads/attachment_data/file/518000/Nursing_and_Midwifery_Amendment_Order_2016_Draft_A.pdf (accessed 3 April 2019)

Nursing and Midwifery Council (2014) *Standards for Competence for Registered Nurses.* London: NMC.

Nursing and Midwifery Council (2018a) *Future Nurse: standards of proficiency for registered nurses.* London: NMC.

Nursing and Midwifery Council (2018b) *Realising Professionalism: standards for education and training Part 1: Standards framework for nursing and midwifery education.* London: NMC.

Nursing and Midwifery Council (2018c) *Realising Professionalism: standards for education and training Part 2: Standards for student supervision and assessment.* London: NMC.

Nursing and Midwifery Council (2018d) *Realising Professionalism: standards for education and training Part 3: Standards for pre-registration nursing programmes.* London: NMC.

Nursing and Midwifery Council (2018e) *The Code: professional standards of practice and behaviour for nurses, midwives and nursing associates.* London: NMC.

Royal College of Nursing (2014) *Defining Nursing.* London: RCN.

Royal College of Nursing (2016) Mentorship Project. *From Today's Support in Practice to Tomorrow's Vision for Excellence.* London: RCN.

Royal College of Nursing (2017) *Helping Students Get the Best From Their Practice Placements: a Royal College of Nursing toolkit.* London: RCN.

Useful websites

www.learning-styles-online.com (accessed 3 April 2019)
www.nmc.org.uk (accessed 3 April 2019)

COMMUNICATION

The aim of this chapter is to introduce briefly the concept of communication in the context of healthcare delivery.

LEARNING OUTCOMES

On completion of this chapter you should:
- understand the definitions and the process of communication
- be able to identify and overcome the barriers that may prevent effective communication taking place
- understand the skills required for effective and active listening
- have explored the concept of emotional quotient/intelligence
- understand how nurses are advocates and empower clients
- understand the importance of digital literacy

» Introduction

Communication skills are an essential element of professionalism and an essential element of the NMC (2018) standards of proficiency for registered nurses. In Platform 1 of that document, 'Being an accountable professional', it states that "[Registered nurses] ... communicate effectively, are role models for others and are accountable for their actions." Communication is also one of the 6Cs, as presented in *Chapter 1* and discussed more fully in *Chapter 3*. Consequently as a student nurse you will be required to develop and maintain a high level of intra- and interpersonal communication. In fact it is probably one of the most important skills you will need, wherever your area of practice might be, because you must be able to communicate effectively to provide competent nursing care. Despite this importance, it is well recognised that many practitioners do not always communicate with others as well as they should.

≫ Communication defined

A considerable number of definitions of communication can be found in the literature, such as:

- "The process by which we understand others and in turn endeavour to be understood by them" (McCorry and Mason, 2011).
- "A two-way process of reaching mutual understanding, in which participants not only exchange information but also create and share meaning" (O'Toole, 2016).
- "A complex process of sending and receiving verbal and non-verbal messages that allows for an exchange of information, feelings, needs, preferences and embraces culture" (Kersey-Matusiak, 2013). The concept of culture will influence a person's health and wellbeing and is discussed in *Chapter 5*.
- "In nursing, communication is a sharing of health-related information between a patient and a nurse, with both participants as sources and receivers. The information may be verbal or non-verbal, written or spoken, personal or impersonal, issue-specific or even relationship-orientated" (Sheldon, 2013).

≫ The communication process

One way of beginning to explain how communication occurs is the baseline process model of communication. Based on the work of Shannon and Weaver (1949), this model is still one of the most widely used as a starting point to understand the process of communication.

The communication process is made up of four key components, as shown in *Figure 2.1*.

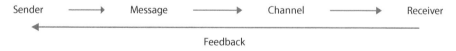

Figure 2.1: *A process model of communication.*

The sender (transmitter)

The sender is an individual, group or organisation that initiates the communication. All communication begins with the sender and the source is initially responsible for the success of the message. The first step for the sender involves the encoding process.

The message

In order to convey meaning the sender must translate (encode) information into a message in the form of symbols that represent ideas, concepts, etc.

These symbols can take numerous forms such as languages, words or gestures. It is clearly important for the sender to use symbols that are familiar to and appropriate for the intended receiver.

The channel

The channel is the means by which the sender conveys the message. Channels or types of communication generally come under the main headings:
- verbal
- non-verbal
- tactile
- written.

The receiver

After the appropriate channel or channels have been selected, the message enters the decoding stage of the communication process. Decoding is conducted by the receiver. Once the message is received, the stimulus is sent to the brain for interpreting in order to assign some type of meaning. The receiver translates the message into their own set of experiences in order to make the symbols meaningful. All interpretations by the receiver are influenced by their experiences, attitudes, knowledge, skills, perceptions and culture (as with the sender's encoding) (Foulger, 2004).

Although, according to this model which is still readily used in current literature, communication is seemingly a simple activity, in reality it is not. It is a complex process in which many other factors need to be considered for effective communication to take place.

≫ Interpersonal skills

Put simply, interpersonal skills are the skills we use to interact or deal with others.

Allender *et al.* (2014) suggest that in nursing there are three particular types of interpersonal skills that build on sending and receiving skills, and these are:
- respect
- rapport
- trust.

Respect

According to Peate (2012, p. 153), respect relates to the ability of a nurse to demonstrate a sincere interest in the patient and his or her needs. Expressing a genuine wish to understand, showing kindness and patience, and being concerned for any fears or discomfort the patient may have, are all ways of demonstrating respect to the patient and their family.

Rapport

Rapport links to showing respect and is about sympathetic and harmonious relationships, especially ones of emotional affinity and mutual trust.

Trust

Trust is about integrity and having faith and confidence in another person. In nursing, Allender *et al.* (2014) suggest that trust is developed by providing an open, honest and patient-focused approach.

Empathy

A further interpersonal skill that is important to mention here is empathy. Definitions of empathy are many but essentially it is about the attempt to understand and share, in a non-judgemental way, the feelings, experiences and concerns of others. Empathy for the most part is a learnt skill or attitude and although it is unlikely that a person who develops such a skill could ever know exactly what another person actually feels, it is important that the nurse should learn to make the attempt to

>> Empathy is essentially the attempt to understand and share the feelings, experiences and concerns of others.

do so. Empathising with a patient, a carer, etc. can only enhance the ability to communicate effectively. Being empathetic means you need to have an intelligent and emotional understanding of the situation the patient and family are going through (Edwards, 2001).

>> Intercultural communication

Cultural competence is a set of attitudes, skills, behaviours and policies that enable people (staff) and organisations to work effectively in cross-cultural situations; this includes intercultural communication skills, as nurses and other healthcare professionals communicate and share information with people from other cultures and social groups. In order to develop cultural competence you need to develop knowledge and awareness, and have a good attitude and appropriate skills (see also *Chapter 5*).

RECAP

- Communication is one of the most important skills you will need because you must be able to communicate effectively to provide competent nursing care.
- Interpersonal skills are the skills we use to interact or deal with others.

ACTIVITY 2.1

Take a few minutes to reflect back on one or two experiences of being involved in caring for someone where you have utilised the interpersonal skills identified above. Think of a situation where you have worked with another person who is not from the same culture as you. Can you think of how you could have improved this interaction?

>> Emotional intelligence

A relatively recent behavioural model linked to communication and interpersonal skills is that of Emotional Intelligence (EI). Emotional intelligence describes an ability to perceive, assess and manage one's own emotions and those of others (Goldman, 2017; Walsh, 2018).

>> People who exhibit a high degree of emotional intelligence tend to be more fulfilled and productive than others in every area of their lives.

The EI concept suggests that IQ (intelligence quotient), the traditional measure of intelligence, is too limiting as it ignores essential behavioural and character elements. EI encompasses the wider areas of intelligence that dictate and contribute to how successful an individual is; an example often used is that of a person who can be academically brilliant and yet socially and interpersonally inept; we know that despite their possessing a high IQ rating, success does not automatically follow.

Essentially EI has two main aspects, namely:
• understanding yourself
• understanding others and their feelings.

Within these aspects there are four key dimensions:
• **Self-awareness** – knowing one's internal states, preferences, goals, intentions, etc.
• **Social awareness** – awareness of the feelings, needs and concerns of others
• **Self-management** – managing one's internal states, impulses and resources to facilitate reaching goals
• **Social skills** – adeptness at inducing desirable responses in others.

Extensive research on the subject appears to suggest that the process and outcomes of EI development contain many elements known to reduce stress for individuals and organisations, by decreasing conflict and improving relationships and understanding. Also, those who exhibit a high degree of EI tend to be more fulfilled and productive than others in every area of their lives: personal, professional and family (Walsh, 2018; Goldman, 2017).

ACTIVITY 2.2

There is a considerable amount of information on the internet relating to emotional intelligence. This includes many sites that provide an opportunity to measure your own level of EI. As a starting point use a general search engine, such as Google, to search for an Emotional Intelligence Test.

>> Non-verbal interaction

Verbal and non-verbal skills are closely interrelated and thus non-verbal interaction in healthcare is also extremely important. Faulkner (1997, p. 76) suggests that, generally, if concurrent verbal and non-verbal messages do not match, then the non-verbal message is the one more likely to be believed.

Non-verbal interaction includes the following:

- **Gesture** – e.g. with hands, arms, head. The gestures people use convey meanings; for example, arms firmly crossed and head turned away can give a negative message to the receiver.
- **Posture** – e.g. sitting, standing, slouching. The way that we stand or sit gives information about how we are feeling; for example, a nurse sitting slumped in a chair can give a negative message.
- **Facial expressions** – our faces can show many of our feelings. For example, a frown or a smile shows a very clear message, depending on how and when it is used.
- **Eye contact** – maintaining appropriate eye contact when speaking with others helps positive communication. Avoiding eye contact may suggest that you do not really want to communicate, or that you may be telling a lie. Although eye contact for several seconds is good, you should also be aware that staring or excessive eye contact may make a person feel uncomfortable.
- **Proximity** – most people feel uncomfortable when somebody stands or sits either too close or too far away from them. When this situation happens, it can make communication more difficult.

There is no doubt that when you focus on combining verbal and non-verbal messages in the most effective way possible, you should significantly improve your overall communication skills.

ACTIVITY 2.3

The next time you interact with a patient, carer, service user, etc., stop and think about your non-verbal communication – what message/s do you think you are conveying to the receiver of your message? Sometimes it is hard to judge ourselves so you might like to ask a trusted friend or family member what they think about your non-verbal messages.

» Barriers to effective communication

Unfortunately there are many ways in which the message being transmitted in the communication process either never reaches the receiver, or fails to be understood or is misinterpreted by the receiver. Such barriers to effective communication include the following:

- Non-verbal:
  - negative messages from body language
- Linguistic:
  - speaking too quickly or too slowly
  - too much or too little information given at one time
  - language differences
  - regional or national accents
  - use of technical jargon
  - restricted or elaborate code of speech
  - level of voice
  - tone of voice
- Cultural:
  - different values, social norms, rules and rituals – this relates to both verbal and non-verbal communication, and can include social class, perceptions and prejudices
- Social:
  - background and education
  - status of the sender – communication is easier if the perceived power differential is low
- Individual/personal:
  - emotional state of the receiver
  - sensory deficits
  - poor cognitive skills
  - fatigue
  - mistrust
  - past experiences
  - need to know – is the information being received important to the receiver or not?

- External/structural:
  - appropriate place for communication (e.g. is privacy required?)
  - noise
  - distractions.

ACTIVITY 2.4

Note down a few key points that you think may help overcome some of the barriers to effective communication listed above.

Overcoming communication barriers

The following are a few points to consider when communicating with service users and their families:

- Select the best location – communicate somewhere that will encourage effective communication.
- Being positive and supportive rather than negative and defensive helps make communication more effective.
- Ensure the best channel for communication has been chosen.
- Be respectful and empathise if appropriate.
- Always be culturally and socially aware with regard to those with whom you are communicating.
- Ensure communication is clear, concise, concrete, correct and courteous.
- Use repetition – repeating messages using different examples or channels can sometimes help the receiver to understand the message being sent.
- Check written communication for spelling errors and ensure the sentences are clear, concise and not ambiguous.
- Develop good listening skills.

(Burnard and Gill, 2009; Peate, 2012; Sheldon, 2013; Kersey-Matusiak, 2013)

>> Listening skills

In healthcare listening is an integral and important part of the communication process. However, it can also be one of the most challenging skills for the nurse to develop. The following can be barriers to effective listening:

- Verbal activities, e.g.:
  - interrupting
  - asking questions at inappropriate times
  - preoccupation with other issues
  - noise

- – individual bias and prejudices
- – hearing only what you want to hear
- – trying to work out what the speaker means rather than listening to what is actually being said
- Non-verbal activities, e.g.:
  - – avoiding eye contact
  - – bored expression, yawning
  - – fiddling and fidgeting
  - – checking watches or phones
  - – tidying papers, etc.
  - – perceived time restriction
  - – inattention generally.

Unfortunately, some of the above activities happen far too frequently in the busy area of healthcare practice.

Good listening skills

Good listening skills are not just about being silent and passively receiving the thoughts and feelings of others. To be an effective listener, you need to respond with verbal and non-verbal cues which communicate to the speaker that you are listening to what they are saying. Good listening skills include:

- Give the speaker your undivided attention and look at the speaker directly (not at what else is going on around you).
- Make sure your mind is focused. If you feel your mind wandering, change the position of your body and try to concentrate on the speaker's words.
- Listen for main ideas. Pay special attention to statements that begin with phrases such as *'My point is...'* or *'The thing to remember is...'*. Also 'listen' to the speaker's non-verbal cues.
- Show you are listening – use body language to convey your attention. For example, nod occasionally, smile and use facial expressions, and ensure your posture is open and welcoming.
- Don't interrupt; let the speaker finish before you begin to talk and let yourself finish listening before you begin to speak. Wait for the right opportunity to ask questions.
- If you are not sure you understand what the speaker has said, you need to check with them to ensure your understanding is correct. This may be achieved by repeating their words (for example, the last few words of the sentence) or by reflecting back in your own words (paraphrasing) what the speaker has said.
- Keep an open and receptive mind to people and their thoughts.
- Be respectful and courteous at all times.

Remember that listening takes time or, more accurately, that you have to take time to listen (Peate, 2012).

RECAP

- Non-verbal interaction in healthcare is very important.
- You need to be aware of the potential barriers to effective communication and ways to overcome them.
- Listening is an integral part of the communication process and it is important to develop good listening skills as a nurse in order to provide effective and compassionate care to your patients.

» Advocacy and empowerment

We hope that by now you understand that part of being a nurse is to be the liaison between patients and doctors or other healthcare professionals, and between patients and their family. This we call being an advocate, as nurses help patients understand their diagnosis and make the best decisions about their health. Empowerment means having the freedom and power to do what you want or to control what happens – an empowered patient feels able to participate in decision-making with healthcare professionals (see also *Chapter 11*). However, sometimes patients are too ill or feel unable to express their feelings and nurses need to help them communicate this and where necessary 'be their voice' as they advocate for the patient. This support means that nurses need to act in the interest of the patient's beliefs and preferences, even if this causes conflict with other healthcare professionals or, potentially, the patient's family.

ACTIVITY 2.5

First, consider what communication skills are necessary when you are advocating for a patient. Secondly, think about how you might help a patient express their needs and concerns and how you can empower them to voice these.

» Digital literacy

More and more aspects of healthcare are electronic, such as vital sign recording, test results, blood tests, ordering medication, etc., and this new healthcare technology is creating opportunities for nurses. There is an array of new technologies used in healthcare today – mobile devices, electronic medical records, cloud computing and teleconferencing – and these are all methods of communication, which means nurses need to be digitally literate. Patients and families are also evolving in a digitalised world as they use online resources to research and treat their symptoms. Consequently, nurses need to be up to date in health technology, trustworthy websites and useful applications (apps) as they direct patients.

ACTIVITY 2.6

Are you digitally literate? What digital sources have you used? How do you know these are trustworthy?

CHAPTER SUMMARY

- The communication process is made up of four key components, i.e. the sender, a message, a channel and the receiver.
- Interpersonal skills are the skills we use to interact or deal with others.
- Emotional intelligence is a behavioural model linked to communication and interpersonal skills and describes the ability to perceive, access and manage one's own emotions and those of others.
- Verbal and non-verbal interaction and skills are closely related, and both are extremely important in healthcare.
- Barriers to effective communication are numerous, therefore an understanding of what they might be and how they might be overcome is critical.
- Listening is an integral part of the communication process. To be an effective listener you need to respond with verbal and non-verbal cues which communicate to the speaker that you are listening.
- Nursing involves being an advocate for patients and empowering them to voice their needs, and a nurse must have good communication skills to enable this.
- 21st-century communication is also embedded within the electronic world and nurses need to be digitally competent.

Further information

- *Communication and Interpersonal Skills*, 2nd edition, by E. Pavord and E. Donnelly (Lantern Publishing, 2015) provides an opportunity to further explore the theory that underpins communication studies and also self-assess your own communication and interpersonal skills.
- *Delivering Culturally Competent Nursing Care* by G. Kersey-Matusiak (Springer, 2013) provides an opportunity for you to explore what cultural competency is.

- *Communication for Nurses: talking with patients*, 3rd edition, by L.K. Sheldon (Jones & Bartlett, 2013) is a comprehensive text which prepares you for a career in healthcare, providing you with the tools necessary to develop a professional communication style. It offers a clear and concise approach to communication development.
- www.mindtools.com contains many resources to help you learn about management, leadership and personal effectiveness skills, including communication.
- www.businessballs.com is a free ethical learning and development resource for people and organisations, and includes resources about emotional intelligence.

References

Allender, J.A., Rector, C. and Warner, K.D. (2014) *Community and Public Health Nursing: promoting the public's health*, 8th edition. Philadelphia, PA: Wolters Kluwer Health.

Burnard, P. and Gill, P. (2009) *Culture, Communication and Nursing*. Abingdon: Routledge.

Edwards, S.D. (2001) *Philosophy of Nursing: an introduction*. Basingstoke: Palgrave.

Faulkner, A. (1997) *Effective Interaction with Patients*, 2nd edition. Edinburgh: Churchill Livingstone.

Foulger, D. (2004) *Models of the Communication Process*. Available at: davis.foulger.info/research/unifiedModelOfCommunication.htm (accessed 4 April 2019)

Goldman, A. (2017) *Emotional Intelligence: why it is more important than IQ and how you can improve yours*. CreateSpace Independent Publishing Platform.

Kersey-Matusiak, G. (2013) *Delivering Culturally Competent Nursing Care*. New York: Springer.

McCorry, L.K. and Mason, J. (2011) *Communication Skills for the Healthcare Professional*. Baltimore, MD: Lippincott Williams & Wilkins.

Nursing and Midwifery Council (2018) *Future Nurse: standards of proficiency for registered nurses*. London: NMC.

O'Toole, G. (2016) *Communication: core interpersonal skills for health professionals*, 3rd edition. Chatswood, NSW: Elsevier.

Peate, I. (2012) *The Student's Guide to Becoming a Nurse*, 2nd edition. Chichester: Wiley-Blackwell.

Shannon, C.E. and Weaver, W. (1949) *The Mathematical Theory of Communication*. Urbana, IL: University of Illinois Press.

Sheldon, L.K. (2013) *Communication for Nurses: talking with patients*, 3rd edition. Burlington, MA: Jones & Bartlett Learning.

Walsh, M. (2018) *Key Topics in Social Sciences: an A–Z guide for student nurses*. Banbury: Lantern Publishing Ltd.

LEGAL AND
PROFESSIONAL ISSUES

The aim of this chapter is to make you aware of the legal and professional issues surrounding nursing.

LEARNING OUTCOMES

On completion of this chapter you should be able to:
- demonstrate an awareness of the legal framework within which care is provided
- discuss the legal responsibilities of nurses when caring for patients or clients
- discuss the nurse's responsibility when using social media
- define the term 'accountability' in relation to *The Code: professional standards of practice and behaviour for nurses, midwives and nursing associates* (NMC, 2018a) and other guidelines issued by the Nursing and Midwifery Council

You may not feel that all the considerations discussed in this chapter apply to you, as you are not yet a Nursing and Midwifery Council (NMC) registrant. However, as a citizen or resident of the United Kingdom (UK) the legal aspects do apply (under both criminal and civil law). In addition you are advised to look on the NMC regulations as a guide for best practice. Any employment regulation may affect you when undertaking clinical practice and you should also be aware of any charters, guidelines, policies, etc. that your university or college and/or placement organisation asks you to respect.

» Accountability

The importance of accountability in professional life is not new, and nurses and student nurses are accountable and must be aware of the implications of this. Accountability is to be liable for what you have, or have not done, and to give an account of your decisions.

Accountability is often defined as responsibility, but there is a difference between the two:

- Responsibility is concerned with answering for what you do, whereas
- Accountability is being answerable for the 'consequences' of what you do.

The most important factor in accountability is that it is 'personal' and no registered nurse can be accountable for another. Before registration you are not *professionally* accountable in the way that you will be after registering with the NMC; however, the NMC states that as a student you must conduct yourself professionally and in alignment with the *Code* (NMC, 2018a).

This chapter explores those legal boundaries.

» Arenas of accountability

As you can see from *Figure 3.1*, Dimond (2015), a barrister who has a great interest in professional accountability and patients' rights, believes there are four arenas of accountability which nurses must consider.

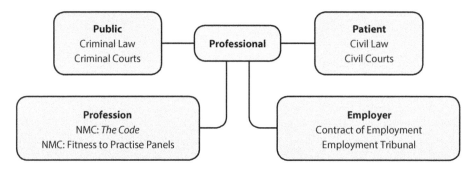

Figure 3.1: *Arenas of accountability (adapted from Dimond, 2015).*

Criminal law and the courts

In criminal law, a crime is committed against the state either when an act is performed that the law forbids, or when an act is omitted that the law requires. For a conviction it must be proved that a person intended to commit the crime, or was reckless in doing the criminal act. More serious cases include murder, manslaughter and rape (all of which nurses have been found guilty of) and are heard in a Crown Court before a judge and jury. Lesser cases (such as driving offences) are heard in a magistrates' court. The outcome of prosecution is a custodial sentence or a fine, or both.

Civil law and the courts

This part of the law involves the rights and duties individuals have towards each other. Legal action can be taken by a private individual against another individual or an organisation. This is the main area which affects nurses and which lawyers refer to as the law of torts. The outcomes from these cases usually involve awards of compensation (for damages) or orders (injunctions) to stop an individual acting unlawfully. The NMC recognises that this is an area where nurses are increasingly being involved and states that nurses must have an indemnity arrangement which provides appropriate cover for their practice (NMC, 2018a, Clause 12.1).

Duty of candour

The professional duty of candour means that every healthcare professional must be open and honest with patients when something goes wrong with their treatment or when care causes, or has the potential to cause, harm or distress (NMC, 2015a). The duty of candour means that healthcare professionals must apologise to the patient (or, where appropriate, the patient's advocate, carer or family) when

>> Every healthcare professional must be open and honest with patients when something goes wrong.

something goes wrong, and if possible offer an appropriate remedy or support to put matters right. This means that the healthcare professional must explain fully the short- and long-term implications of what has happened.

Healthcare professionals must also be open and honest with their colleagues, employers and relevant organisations, and take part in reviews and investigations when requested. They must raise concerns where appropriate and support and encourage each other to be open and honest (NMC, 2015a).

The UK government introduced the Statutory Duty of Candour in 2014, following several high-profile national reports. These include Berwick (2013) – *Improving Patient Safety*, Keogh (2013) – *Review into the Quality of Care and Treatment provided by 14 Hospital Trusts in England* and Francis (2013) – *The Mid Staffordshire NHS Foundation Trust Public Enquiry*, which identified the suffering of many patients within a culture of secrecy and defensiveness.

Francis (2013) also highlighted a whole system failure which should have had checks and balances in place, to ensure that patients were treated with dignity and suffered no harm. The report called for a "fundamental change" in culture whereby patients are put first, and it made a total of 290 recommendations covering a broad range of issues relating to patient care and safety in the NHS. These detailed recommendations did not call for a reorganisation of the system but rather a re-emphasis on what is important, at all levels of health service in England, to try to prevent such problems happening again.

The Statutory Duty of Candour was introduced for Trusts, Foundation Trusts, special health authorities and all other providers registered with the Care Quality Commission (CQC). The aim of the duty is to provide a much more open and transparent healthcare system, and to improve safety in the NHS. Directors of healthcare settings are not only responsible for the overall quality, safety and care of their patients, but also for ensuring every healthcare professional is open and honest with patients when something goes wrong with their treatment or care, or has the potential to cause harm or distress. In addition, healthcare professionals must be open and honest with their colleagues, employers and relevant organisations and take part in reviews and investigations when requested.

The NMC has also emphasised the need for nurses and midwives to abide by their Duty of Candour within the *Code* (NMC, 2018a, Section 14): "Be open and candid with all service users about all aspects of care and treatment, including when any mistakes or harm have taken place."

Freedom to speak up: raising concerns (whistleblowing) policy for the NHS (NHSI, 2016)

This policy was developed from recommendations of the review by Sir Robert Francis into whistleblowing in the NHS. The government expects the policy to be adopted, "as a minimum standard, by all NHS organisations, in England to help normalise the raising of concerns for the benefit of patients" (NHSI, 2016, p. 3). Concerns about risk, malpractice, or wrongdoing can be raised openly, confidentially or anonymously by anyone who works (or has worked) in the NHS or for an independent organisation that provides NHS services, in person, by phone or in writing (including email).

As a student nurse, if you have any doubts about the actions or performance of a registered nurse, you must not ignore the situation even if it could put you in a difficult position. The *Code* (NMC, 2018a, Clause 16.1) advises that you "raise and, if necessary, escalate any concerns you may have about patient or public safety, or the level of care people are receiving in your workplace or any other health and care setting and use the channels available to you in line with our guidance and your local working practices". You will find that your higher education establishment has a Raising Concerns Policy and this guides you regarding how to raise a concern and the processes and support you will be offered during this process; your university advisor will help you.

A concern may be raised internally, either informally or formally with a line manager (or lead clinician or tutor/lecturer). If this is not deemed appropriate by the individual(s) reporting a concern it may be raised with any of the following:

- A designated Freedom to Speak up Guardian (FTSU) (or equivalent designated person) – the FTSU acts as an independent and impartial source of advice with direct and regular access to members of Trust boards and other senior leaders
- The organisation's risk management team
- The executive or non-executive director with responsibility for whistleblowing within the organisation
- Externally with relevant organisations, e.g. the CQC.

On receipt, the concern is recorded and the individual(s) will receive an acknowledgement of this within two working days. Issues of confidentiality will be noted at this time. Following this, any concerns not able to be resolved quickly through the line manager should be proportionately investigated. Investigations are expected to be evidence-based and led by someone suitably independent in the organisation who is also required to produce a report which focuses on learning lessons and improving care. Individuals should be kept informed throughout of the investigation's progress (NHS Improvement, 2018).

Duty of care (negligence)

An action for negligence is a civil action, and results from a breach of duty of care. A nurse may be held legally liable if it can be shown that they have either failed to exercise the skills properly expected of them, or undertaken tasks that they are not competent to perform (Dimond, 2015).

For negligence to be proved, the following conditions must be satisfied:
1. A duty of care is owed by the defendant (nurse) to the claimant (patient), i.e. the nurse–patient relationship (duty)
2. There is a breach in the standard of care owed (breach)
3. This breach has caused reasonably foreseeable harm (causation)
4. This breach has caused harm, either by action or omission.

Some criminal cases may also have a civil action brought if any harm has been caused by 'action or omission'.

ACTIVITY 3.1

Think of a circumstance where a nurse might be held criminally liable (i.e. a criminal act that a nurse might commit).

Think of circumstances in clinical practice where a nurse might be judged negligent (i.e. perform an act that could be referred to a civil court).

Accountability to the employer

Everyone in a nursing role is accountable to their employer. There is an implied term in every contract of employment that the employee will obey the reasonable instructions of the employer (i.e. follow any policies, procedures, standards, etc.), and that any employee who breaches their contract may be subject to disciplinary action. Even though, as a student nurse, you are not 'employed' by a placement organisation as such, you are still bound by their

>> As a student nurse, you are bound by the reasonable instructions of your placement providers.

'instructions', and any deviation from these could lead to disciplinary action by your university and/or your placement provider. You must therefore be familiar with the policies, procedures, etc. of your placement provider, as you could be called to account by your university or by the law.

Vicarious liability

An employer is liable for any actions committed by their employees (for example nurses) during the scope of their employment. The employer (for example, an NHS Trust or a care home) cannot shirk this liability by saying they provide competent, trained staff – they will always be primarily responsible for any negligence to patients by their staff (Dimond, 2015).

However, this does not remove any legal responsibility/accountability from the nurse. If a patient takes a civil action against a hospital (for example, for damages caused by one of its employees), and the hospital is found directly liable by the civil courts, the hospital as the employer could in turn take legal action against the employee. This usually happens when a hospital (an employer) has to pay compensation to a patient as a result of an employee's negligence, and tries to recoup their money from the employee. As this falls in the arena of civil law, which applies to all citizens and residents of the UK, this could affect you as a student nurse.

FURTHER READING

Further information relating to *No Secrets: guidance on protecting vulnerable adults in care* (Department of Health, 2000) is available at: www.gov.uk/government/publications/ no-secrets-guidance-on-protecting-vulnerable-adults-in-care

---

Professional liability – the Nursing and Midwifery Council

The core function of the NMC is to establish standards of education, training, conduct and performance for nursing and midwifery and to ensure those standards are maintained, thereby safeguarding the health and wellbeing of the public. The powers of the NMC are set out in the Nursing and Midwifery

(Amendment) Order 2016. Although you are a student nurse, you are already affected by the role of the NMC as it sets the standards of education and training you are undertaking. The NMC determines the level of entry and content of pre-registration nursing programmes, and universities have to have validation from the NMC to run such programmes. Programmes are also monitored and reviewed by the NMC on a regular basis, as discussed in *Chapter 1*.

The key responsibilities of the NMC (NMC, 2018b) are to:

- regulate nurses and midwives in England, Wales, Scotland and Northern Ireland
- protect the public
- set standards of education and training
- set standards of conduct and performance so that nurses and midwives can deliver high quality healthcare throughout their careers
- ensure that nurses and midwives keep their skills and knowledge up to date and uphold its professional standards
- give clear and transparent processes to investigate nurses and midwives who fall short of its standards
- maintain a register of nurses and midwives allowed to practise in the UK.

All nurses working in a registered nurse capacity must be registered with the NMC. When you have successfully completed your nursing programme your university will notify the NMC that you have met the required standards and that you are eligible for entry on the register. The NMC requires you to complete a Declaration of Good Health and Good Character before registration can take place (NMC, 2019).

What constitutes good health and good character?

Good health and good character are fundamental to fitness to practise as a nurse.

Good health means that you must be capable of safe and effective practice without supervision. It does not mean the absence of any disability or health condition. Many disabled people and those with health conditions are able to practise, with or without adjustments to support their practice.

Long-term conditions such as epilepsy, diabetes or depression can be well managed and would not be incompatible with registration. Equally, temporary health conditions do not necessarily mean a person is not fit to practise. For example, having a broken leg may mean a person is not fit to work for a period of time. It does not mean they are not fit to practise, as they can reasonably expect to recover fully and return to work.

Good character is important because nurses and midwives must be honest and trustworthy. Your good character is based on your conduct, behaviour and attitude. It covers examples such as someone who knowingly practises as a nurse before they are on the register, or someone who signs a student off from an educational programme while being aware of poor behaviour.

It also includes any convictions and cautions that are not considered compatible with professional registration and that might bring the profession into disrepute. Your character must be sufficiently good for you to be capable of safe and effective practice without supervision (NMC, 2018a and NMC, 2015).

The Code: professional standards of practice and behaviour for nurses, midwives and nursing associates *(NMC, 2018a)*

You must be aware of the professional accountability you will automatically assume once registered. The NMC stresses the need for all registered nurses to be personally accountable for their practice by issuing them with the *Code* (NMC, 2018a). Although this document is not part of law, the functions of the NMC include a requirement to establish and improve standards of professional conduct (Health Act, 2006; Nursing and Midwifery (Amendment) Order, 2016). They do this by issuing the *Code* (NMC, 2018a) and a requirement for all registered nurses to abide by it. Breaching the *Code* is in effect a breach of registration and may lead to the removal of the nurse's name from the register.

>> As a student nurse you are bound by the NMC *Code*.

Paramount in the *Code* is the requirement for registered nurses to have "the knowledge and skills ... for safe and effective practice" (NMC, 2018a, Clause 6.2). In line with this, the NMC warns that careful consideration must be made of professional accountability if nurses are asked to work in an area for which they are not adequately prepared – being open about their limitations is not a sign of weakness but rather a key indicator of mature and caring practice (Peate, 2016).

The *Code* (NMC, 2018a) is divided into four themes with a number of sections under each theme:
• Prioritise people
• Practise effectively
• Preserve safety
• Promote professionalism and trust.

This code of conduct should be considered together with the Nursing and Midwifery Council's rules, standards, guidance and advice, and is available from www.nmc.org.uk.

The NMC acknowledges that as a student you will come into close contact with patients, by observing care being given, by helping to provide care and, towards the end of your course, through full participation in providing care. As a student nurse you are also bound by the *Code* and must conduct yourself professionally at all times. Additionally, the NMC emphasises that you must "raise your concerns immediately if you are being asked to practise beyond your role, experience and training" (NMC, 2018a, Clause 16.2); and "ask for help from a suitably qualified and experienced professional to carry out any action or procedure that is beyond the limits of your competence" (NMC, 2018a, Clause 13.3).

Adherence to the *Code* is important not just in the clinical setting, but also in your university or college. In addition, most universities will ask you to sign a Code or Charter which would include expectations that you would:
- take responsibility for your own learning
- follow the policy on attendance as set out by your university and clinical placement provider
- follow the policy on submission of coursework and completion of clinical assessments as set out by your university and clinical placement provider
- reflect on and respond constructively to feedback you are given
- endeavour to provide care based on the best available evidence or best practice
- not plagiarise or falsify coursework or clinical assessments.

Guidance on the use of social media

The NMC has issued guidelines for all nurses – registered and students – when using social media (NMC, 2015). It recognises that if used responsibly and appropriately, social networking sites can offer benefits, and has acknowledged this in the *Code* (NMC, 2018a, p. 19). However, inappropriate use of social media may put nurses' registration at risk if they act in any way that is unprofessional or unlawful. This equally applies to student nurses, who may be withdrawn from their pre-registration programme.

Examples of inappropriate use include (but are not limited to):
- sharing confidential information inappropriately
- posting pictures of patients and people receiving care without their consent
- posting inappropriate comments about patients
- discussing placement area, practice assessor or staff
- bullying, intimidating or exploiting people
- building or pursuing relationships with patients or service users
- stealing personal information or using someone else's identity
- encouraging violence or self-harm
- inciting hatred or discrimination.

Providing care in an emergency situation outside the work environment

In the UK there is generally no legal obligation to provide care or assistance in an emergency situation. However, in an emergency, in or outside the work setting, registered nurses have a professional duty to provide care, and in providing that care they are accountable for any actions or omissions in their practice, and would be judged against what could reasonably be expected from someone with their knowledge, skills and abilities in those circumstances. They would need to ensure that they work within the limits of their competence and that they are able to demonstrate that they acted in the person's best interests.

The NMC (2018a) has a section (Section 15) on offering help if an emergency arises in your practice setting or anywhere else. It states that you should:

- *"only act in an emergency within the limits of your knowledge and competence* [Clause 15.1]
- *arrange, wherever possible, for emergency care to be accessed and provided promptly* [Clause 15.2]
- *take account of your own safety, the safety of others and the availability of other options for providing care* [Clause 15.3]."

Giving assistance in an emergency or accident spans all the areas of accountability nurses are concerned with (criminal, civil, employment and professional law), and as a student you should be aware of the implications for you.

RECAP

- Accountability is being answerable for the 'consequences' of what you do.
- The four arenas of accountability are the public, the patient, the employer and the profession.
- As a student nurse you are bound by the NMC *Code*. When you qualify you will register and also become professionally accountable to the NMC.

» Disclosure and Barring Service (DBS)

Disclosure

The Disclosure and Barring Service (DBS) helps employers make safer recruitment decisions and prevent unsuitable people from working with vulnerable groups, including children. The DBS searches police records and, where relevant, Barred List information and then issues a DBS certificate to an applicant and employer. The checking service currently offers two levels of DBS check – standard and enhanced.

Referrals

Referrals are made to the DBS when an employer or an organisation has a concern that a person has caused harm or poses a future risk of harm to vulnerable groups. A wide range of employers and organisations are required or empowered to make referrals and these include Trusts, the General Medical Council and the Nursing and Midwifery Council.

Barring

The Barred Lists are a database of people barred from working with children or vulnerable adults. These two lists provide a record of individuals who will not be permitted to work in regulated activity with children and/or vulnerable adults.

The DBS considers a range of information from the police and referrals from employers, regulatory bodies and other agencies as part of a specifically developed decision-making process on whether to include a person on a list.

The DBS will not remove a bar unless it is satisfied that the individual does not pose a risk of harm to children or vulnerable adults. For information on the DBS visit www.gov.uk/government/organisations/disclosure-and-barring-service.

>> *Compassion in Practice*

Prior to the revision of the NMC *Code* (NMC, 2018a) which is partly based on the findings of the Francis Report (2013; see also *Chapter 6*), the Chief Nursing Officer, Jane Cummings (as stated in *Chapter 1*) launched *Compassion in Practice*. Cummings recognised that the context for healthcare and support is changing and challenging, but that patients must receive high quality, compassionate care to achieve excellent health and wellbeing outcomes. The document outlined six fundamental values that underpin compassion in practice; these are known as the '6Cs' and have been reviewed since they were launched (Department of Health, 2016).

The 6Cs

These focus on putting the person being cared for at the heart of the care they are given:

Care

Care is our core business and that of our organisations, and the care we deliver helps the individual person and improves the health of the whole community. Caring defines us and our work. People receiving care expect it to be right for them, consistently, throughout every stage of their life.

Compassion

Compassion is how care is given through relationships based on empathy, respect and dignity – it can also be described as intelligent kindness, and is central to how people perceive their care.

Competence

Competence means all those in caring roles must have the ability to understand an individual's health and social needs and the expertise, clinical and technical knowledge to deliver effective care and treatments based on research and evidence.

Communication

Communication is central to successful caring relationships and to effective teamworking. Listening is as important as what we say and do and essential for "no decision about me, without me". Communication is the key to a good workplace, with benefits for those in our care and staff alike.

Courage

Courage enables us to do the right thing for the people we care for, to speak up when we have concerns and to have the personal strength and vision to innovate and to embrace new ways of working.

Commitment

A commitment to our patients and populations is a cornerstone of what we do. We need to build on our commitment to improve the care and experience of our patients, to take action to make this vision and strategy a reality for all and meet the health, care and support challenges ahead.

FURTHER READING

Compassion in Practice: two years on (Department of Health, 2016). Available at: www.england.nhs.uk/wp-content/uploads/2016/05/cip-two-years-on.pdf

Leading Change, Adding Value (NHS England, 2016). Available at: https://www.england.nhs.uk/leadingchange/about/understanding-lcav/

Liberating the NHS: no decision about me, without me (Department of Health, 2012). Available at: https://assets.publishing.service.gov.uk/government/uploads/system/uploads/attachment_data/file/216980/Liberating-the-NHS-No-decision-about-me-without-me-Government-response.pdf

NHS England also publishes its key priorities; see: www.england.nhs.uk/wp-content/uploads/2017/03/NEXT-STEPS-ON-THE-NHS-FIVE-YEAR-FORWARD-VIEW.pdf

---

» Delegation

Although all registered nurses are personally accountable for their practice, there are instances where nurses are given delegated tasks and delegate tasks themselves.

The NMC has a section in the *Code* (NMC, 2018a, Section 11) outlining the considerations nurses must take before delegating:

- *"only delegate tasks and duties that are within the other person's scope of competence, making sure they fully understand your instructions*
- *make sure that everyone you delegate tasks to is adequately supervised and supported so they can provide safe and compassionate care*
- *confirm that the outcome of any task you have delegated to someone else meets the required standard"*

This second point (Clause 11.2) could affect you if you believe that a registered nurse has delegated you a task and is not supporting or supervising you. As mentioned before, as a student you must recognise and stay within the limits of your competence and work only under the supervision and support of a qualified professional, asking for help from your practice assessor or tutor/lecturer when you need it.

Peate (2012) reminds registered nurses of the legal perspective of delegation, and believes that when delegating a task, the following must be borne in mind:
- When working as a team member you are personally accountable for your own actions or omissions – there is no such concept as team negligence. If harm occurs, you are individually accountable.
- You must make it known and obtain help and supervision from a competent practitioner if you feel an aspect of practice lies beyond your level of competence or outside your area of registration.

» The *Code* in more detail

As previously identified, the *Code* (NMC, 2018a) is divided into sections. The following pages look in more detail at some of the issues the *Code* raises; namely consent, safeguarding, confidentiality and record-keeping.

» Consent

Every mentally competent adult has the right in law to consent to any touching of their person, or to refuse any examination or treatment. If they are touched without consent or other lawful justification, then that person has the right to bring a criminal action for battery, or a civil action for trespass to the person (Dimond, 2015). Furthermore, should harm occur to the patient, it could result in a legal action

> » You must make sure that you get informed consent and document it before carrying out any nursing action or intervention.

against the nurse for negligence. Consent also affirms the person's right to self-determination and autonomy (Caulfield, 2005). Lord Donaldson, once the second most senior judge in England and Wales, pointed out that consent is twofold – first to obtain 'legal' justification for care (as above), and secondly 'clinical' consent to secure the patient's trust and cooperation.

The NMC *Code* states that you must make sure that you get informed consent and document it before carrying out any action (NMC, 2018a, Clause 4.2), and that any information you give a patient so that they can make an informed decision should be accurate and truthful and presented in such a way as to be easily understood.

Consent can be written, verbal or implied ('by cooperation'). They are all equally valid. However, they vary considerably in their value as evidence in proving that consent was given. Consent in writing is the best form of evidence and therefore is the preferred method for patients when any procedure involving some risk is contemplated. As a student you would not be expected to give information to patients about their condition or treatment or to obtain any written consent. However, any form of nursing intervention requires the patient's consent and it is good practice to:

- make sure people know that you are a student
- ensure that you gain their consent before you begin to provide care
- respect the right for people to request care to be provided by a registered professional.

It is a basic principle of law in this country that a mentally competent adult has the right to refuse treatment and take his or her own discharge contrary to medical advice. The NMC (2018a, Clause 4.1) supports this by stating that you must "balance the need to act in the best interests of people at all times with the requirement to respect a person's right to accept or refuse treatment".

Consent must be:

- given by a legally competent person
- informed
- given freely.

A legally competent person

The person giving consent must have the capacity to do so. A legally competent person must be able to understand and retain information and use the information to make an informed decision. You must presume that a patient is competent unless otherwise assessed by a suitably qualified practitioner. The assessment of whether an adult lacks the capacity to consent is made by the clinician providing treatment or care, but it should involve nurses' views as well.

No one has the right to consent on behalf of another competent adult. Further, it is accepted that adults over the age of 16 have the relevant capacity to understand and make their own decisions about medical and nursing treatment (Caulfield, 2005).

Adults temporarily unable to consent

In emergency situations where an adult becomes unable to consent (for example, if they are unconscious), the law allows treatment as long as it is 'in the patient's best interests'. Medical intervention that can be delayed until the patient can consent should be delayed (exceptions to this are if the person has issued an advance directive refusing treatment, in which case the treatment is not given). 'In the patient's best interests' is said to be when a body of other similar treatment providers would also give the same treatment (Tingle and Cribb, 2013), and arises from a court case in 1989 (*F. v. West Berkshire Health Authority*).

Informed consent

The patient must be able to give informed consent to the proposed treatments, and the information given by any healthcare professional (including registered nurses) should include any material risks such as the nature and consequences of the proposed treatment, the consequences of not having the treatment and any alternatives to the treatment.

Given freely

Consent must be given freely – this means that no threats or implied threats must be used, that no 'coercion and undue influence' are applied. Coercion invalidates consent, and if a nurse feels that the patient is being coerced, either by another healthcare professional or by a family member, they should seek to see the patient alone to ascertain that *their* wishes are being adhered to (Peate, 2012).

⟩⟩ Safeguarding

Safeguarding means protecting people's health, wellbeing and human rights, and enabling them to live free from harm, abuse and neglect. It is fundamental to high quality health and social care (CQC, 2018). Safeguarding is not only for children and young people but also for those who lack mental capacity and these groups will be explored further now. The NMC's (2018b) *Standards of proficiency for registered nurses: Assessing Needs and Planning care* 3.9: state that a nurse must "recognise and assess people at risk of harm and the situations that may put them at risk, ensuring prompt action is taken to safeguard those who are vulnerable".

> ⟩⟩ Safeguarding is fundamental to high quality health and social care.

Children and young people

If the patient is under 18 years old (age of consent) the rules concerning consent for medical treatment are different. A person aged 16–17 is allowed to consent to treatment under the Family Law Reform Act (1969), in a similar way to an adult. However, *refusal* of treatment can be overridden by a person with parental authority or a court order until the patient is 18 years old.

A person under the age of 16 years, who has sufficient understanding and intelligence to enable them to understand the proposed treatment or investigation *may* have the capacity to consent (Department of Health, 2009). Children who have these capacities are said to be 'Gillick competent'. The term Gillick (sometimes referred to as 'Fraser' after the judge who heard the case) comes from a court case in 1985 which concerned a teenage girl's right to consent to medical treatment without her parents' knowledge (*Gillick* v. *West Norfolk and Wisbech Area Health Authority*).

An assessment to determine whether a minor is Gillick (Fraser) competent must consider the following questions (Peate, 2012, p. 75):
- Does the child understand the proposed treatment, their medical condition, and the consequences that may emerge if they refuse or agree to treatment?
- Do they understand the moral, social and family issues involved in the decision they are to make?
- Does the mental state of the child fluctuate?
- What treatment is to be performed? Does the child understand the complexities of the proposed treatment and the potential risks associated with it?

Mental Capacity Act (2007)

The Mental Capacity Act affects people living in England and Wales over the age of 16. It is concerned with protecting people who lack the capacity to make their own decisions about a variety of health and social circumstances.

The Act includes:
- a test to determine 'a person's best interests'
- Lasting Powers of Attorney that extend to a person's health and welfare as well as property and money
- a Court of Protection and an office of Public Guardian to support the Court
- deputies who can make decisions in the 'person's best interests'
- a criminal offence of ill-treatment and neglect
- regulation of advance decisions to refuse treatment
- regulation of research in relation to individuals who lack mental capacity

- an Independent Mental Capacity Advocate (IMCA) service for people with no family or friends
- a Code of Practice to accompany the Act – healthcare professionals have a duty to abide by the *Code* (NMC, 2018a).

Underlying principles of the Mental Capacity Act (2007)

- A presumption of capacity: everyone has the right to make their own decisions, so a person must be assumed to have capacity unless it is established that they lack capacity.
- Individuals should be supported where possible so that they can make their own decisions: a person must not be treated as being unable to make a decision unless all practicable steps to help them to do so have been taken, without success.
- People have the right to make decisions which may seem eccentric or unwise to other people: a person is not to be treated as unable to make a clear decision merely because they make an unwise decision.
- Best interests: acts done or decisions made on behalf of a person established to be lacking capacity must be in their best interests.
- Rights and freedoms must be restricted as little as possible: before doing an act or taking a decision on behalf of a person, regard must be had as to whether the purpose underlying that act or decision can be achieved in a way that is less restrictive of their rights or freedom of action.

Deprivation of Liberty Safeguards (DoLS)

The Deprivation of Liberty Safeguards (DoLS) are part of the Mental Capacity Act (2007). The DoLS aim to protect people who lack mental capacity, but who need to be deprived of liberty so they can be given care and treatment in a hospital or care home. They also aim to make sure that people in care homes, hospitals and supported living are looked after in a way that does not inappropriately restrict their freedom.

The safeguards apply to vulnerable people aged 18 or over who have a mental health condition (this includes dementia), who are in hospitals, care homes and supported living, and who do not have the mental capacity (ability) to make decisions about their care or treatment.

The Mental Capacity Act (2007) says that someone who lacks mental capacity cannot do one or more of the following four things:
- understand information given to them
- retain that information long enough to be able to make a decision

- weigh up the information available and understand the consequences of the decision
- communicate their decision – this could be by any possible means, such as talking, using sign language or even simple muscle movements such as blinking an eye or squeezing a hand.

The key elements of the safeguards are:
- to provide the person with a representative
- to give the person (or their representative) the right to challenge a deprivation of liberty through the Court of Protection
- to provide a mechanism for deprivation of liberty to be reviewed and monitored regularly.

These safeguards do not apply when someone is detained ('sectioned') under the Mental Health Act (2007).

Any assessment must be made by at least two assessors – a best interests assessor and a mental health assessor, neither of whom is involved in that person's care or in making any decisions about it. The best interests assessor will be a qualified social worker, nurse, occupational therapist or chartered psychologist with the appropriate training and experience. The mental health assessor must be a doctor (likely to be a psychiatrist or geriatrician). If the assessment determines that a deprivation of liberty would be in the person's best interests, the Local Authority (in England) will grant an authorisation.

Everyone who is subject to an authorised deprivation of liberty must have a 'relevant person's representative' to speak for them. The representative is appointed by the supervisory body authorising the deprivation. Often it will be a family member or friend, or other carer, and they would normally have been involved in the assessment. The representative can gain access to documents about the decision and ask for a review of the decision, and should be informed if anything changes.

If the person has no immediate family or non-professional carer to support them, the supervisory body will appoint a representative. This may be an independent mental capacity advocate (IMCA). The representative must stay in touch with the person deprived of their liberty in order to fulfil their role and to protect the rights of that person.

There have been several test cases in the European Court of Human Rights and in the UK that have clarified which situations may constitute a deprivation of liberty:
- a patient being restrained in order to admit them to hospital
- medication being given against a person's will
- staff having complete control over a patient's care or movements for a long period

- staff making all decisions about a patient, including choices about assessments, treatment and visitors
- staff deciding whether a patient can be released into the care of others or to live elsewhere
- staff refusing to discharge a person into the care of others
- staff restricting a person's access to their friends or family.

(www.alzheimers.org.uk)

FURTHER READING

Mental Capacity and Deprivation of Liberty (Law Commission, 2017). Available at: www.lawcom.gov.uk/project/mental-capacity-and-deprivation-of-liberty/

Guidance on the safeguards can be found at: www.gov.uk/government/publications/ deprivation-of-liberty-safeguards-forms-and-guidance

Deprivation of Liberty Safeguards (DoLS) at a glance (Social Care Institute of Excellence, 2017). Available at: www.scie.org.uk/mca/dols/at-a-glance

---

Advance decisions to refuse treatment

The Mental Capacity Act (2007) allows adults over the age of 18 years to state, in writing, in advance, what treatment they would *not* like carried out, should they become unable to give consent. These decisions must be respected by all healthcare professionals, including nurses. The person must be deemed competent when making the advance directive, and only clear refusals of specific treatments will be upheld (surgery, drug therapy, etc.).

If any doubt exists, then treatment may be given 'in the patient's best interests'. Furthermore, a patient cannot refuse basic care, but if treatment falls within the remit of the Mental Health Act 2007, refusal cannot be overridden by an advance directive (Peate, 2012).

Mental Health Acts

For people detained under relevant mental health legislation, the principles of consent continue to apply for all conditions not related to the mental disorder.

FURTHER READING

Mental Health Act 2007 – Overview: http://webarchive.nationalarchives.gov.uk/+/http:// www.dh.gov.uk/en/Healthcare/Mentalhealth/DH_078743

➤➤ Confidentiality

Confidentiality is a fundamental part of the patient–carer relationship. Any information given to a nurse by a patient should not be passed on to anyone outside the healthcare team without the patient's consent. The fundamental importance of trust between a health professional and the patient brings with it a 'duty of confidence' (Caulfield, 2005).

This duty arises from:

- duty of care in negligence (discussed earlier in the chapter) – a breach of confidentiality can lead to civil action
- implied duties under the nurse's contract of employment
- requirements of the NMC outlined in the *Code* – a breach of this could result in removal from the nurses' register.

The NMC endorses Caulfield's statements in the *Code* by stating (NMC, 2018a, Section 5): "As a nurse, midwife or nursing associate, you owe a duty of confidentiality to all those who are receiving care. This includes making sure that they are informed about their care and that information about them is shared appropriately."

Disclosing information

Although the *Code* requires you to respect patient confidentiality, it also states that you must share information if you believe someone may be at risk of harm, in line with the laws relating to the disclosure of information (NMC 2018a, Clause 17.2).

However, disclosure of confidential information without consent should only happen in exceptional circumstances. Nurses must be able to justify their actions in doing so, and it must only be done in the public interest to protect individuals, groups or society as a whole from the risk of significant harm. Examples could include child abuse, serious crime or drug trafficking. If a decision to disclose is made, a clear and accurate account should be recorded in the person's records.

Dimond (2015) summarises this when stating that there are seven exceptions to the duty of confidence, when nurses can divulge information about their patients:

- with the patient's consent
- in the patient's best interests
- by court order
- under a statutory duty to disclose
- in the public interests
- to the police
- under provisions within the EU's General Data Protection Regulation (GDPR) (European Parliament, 2016), which replaced the Data Protection Act (1998), because it is a framework with greater scope and has tough punishments for those who fail to comply with new rules around the storage and handling of personal data.

Confidentiality does not only apply within a healthcare setting. As a student you may wish to refer to a real-life situation you have been involved with in an academic assignment. If so, your university will have guidelines on confidentiality that you must abide by, which will advise you not to provide any information that could identify a particular patient, or name a specific health or social care area.

Ownership of and access to records

Records of information belong to an organisation (for example, a hospital) and not to specific people. People can, however, request to see their notes, whether on paper and held on a computer (usually on payment of a fee), under the following Acts:

- The Data Protection Act (1998), now superseded by the EU's General Data Protection Regulation (2016), gave the patient statutory rights to access personal information in the form of health records held on them (both computer and manually-held records). The definition of 'health record' includes all records relating to their health, such as nursing records, physiotherapy records, laboratory results, etc. The patient also has the right of rectification; that is, correcting or amending the data recorded, if it appears to be inaccurate.
- The Access to Medical Reports Act (1988) gives an individual the right of access to any medical report relating to them which is supplied for employment or insurance purposes.
- The Access to Health Records Act (1990) governs access to health records of deceased people.
- The Freedom of Information Act (2014) and Freedom of Information (Scotland) Act (2002) grant anyone the right to information held by public authorities that is not covered by the Data Protection Act (1998). (All Acts of Parliament can be found on www.legislation.gov.uk.)

Caldicott Guardians

A review was commissioned in 1997 by the Chief Medical Officer of England in response to concerns about protection of patient information, and confidentiality thereof. As a result every NHS organisation is required to appoint a 'Caldicott Guardian' who is responsible for agreeing and reviewing internal protocols governing the protection and use of patient-identifiable information by the staff of their organisations. A helpful manual is available (UK Caldicott Guardian Council, 2017).

ACTIVITY 3.2

Explore what is expected of a Caldicott Guardian at: www.gov.uk/government/uploads/system/uploads/attachment_data/file/581213/cgmanual.pdf

» Record-keeping

Record-keeping is part of the professional duty of care owed by the registered nurse to the patient. As a student you will need to take part in record-keeping activities, provided you have the knowledge and skills to undertake this and you are adequately supervised. Your ability to contribute to record-keeping will be assessed in your practice area by the person delegating the task to you (usually your practice assessor) – they will need to countersign any entries made by you.

> » Record-keeping is an integral part of nursing and midwifery practice.

Record-keeping is an integral part of nursing and midwifery practice. It is a tool of professional practice and one that should help the care process, and it is not an optional extra to be fitted in if circumstances allow. Failure to maintain reasonable standards of record-keeping could be evidence of professional misconduct and subject to professional conduct proceedings. Record-keeping is covered within the *Code* (NMC, 2018a, Section 10): "Keep clear and accurate records relevant to your practice".

This includes, but is not limited to patient records. It includes all records that are relevant to your scope of practice.

To achieve this, you must:

> *"10.1 complete records at the time or as soon as possible after an event, recording if the notes are written some time after the event*
>
> *10.2 identify any risks or problems that have arisen and the steps taken to deal with them, so that colleagues who use the records have all the information they need*
>
> *10.3 complete records accurately and without any falsification, taking immediate and appropriate action if you become aware that someone has not kept to these requirements*
>
> *10.4 attribute any entries you make in any paper or electronic records to yourself, making sure they are clearly written, dated and timed, and do not include unnecessary abbreviations, jargon or speculation*

10.5 take all steps to make sure that records are kept securely

10.6 collect, treat and store all data and research findings appropriately."

(NMC, 2018a)

The *Code* (NMC, 2018a) emphasises the need for good record-keeping to protect the welfare of patients/clients by:
- helping to improve accountability
- showing how decisions related to patient care were made
- supporting the delivery of services
- supporting effective clinical judgements and decisions
- supporting patient care and communications
- making continuity of care easier
- providing documentary evidence of services delivered
- promoting better communication and sharing of information between members of the multi-professional healthcare team
- helping to identify risks, and enabling early detection of complications
- supporting clinical audit, research, allocation of resources and performance planning
- helping to address complaints or legal processes.

Patients should be equal partners, whenever possible, in the completion of their records. They have the right to expect that all healthcare professionals will practise a high standard of record-keeping. Therefore, failure on the part of a nurse to maintain reasonable standards of record-keeping could be evidence of professional misconduct and subject to Fitness to Practise proceedings. Records can also be called as evidence by the Health Services Commissioner, before a court of law, or in a local investigation of a complaint made by a patient. This may include anything that makes reference to a patient, such as:
- handwritten medical/nursing notes
- emails
- letters to and from other healthcare professionals
- laboratory reports
- X-rays
- printouts from monitoring equipment
- incident reports and statements
- photographs
- videos
- recordings of telephone conversations
- text messages
- electronic records
- social media.

Any absence of a record may be seen as a lack of care, negligence, inability to write a record, lack of interest, concealment or a general failure to communicate in the best interest of the patient. The ability to write down observations is vital if a nurse needs to testify in court.

Content and style

The principles of good record-keeping include:
- Handwriting should be legible.
- All entries to records should be signed. In the case of written records, the person's name and job title should be printed alongside the first entry.
- In line with local policy, you should put the date and time on all records. This should be in real time and chronological order, and be as close to the actual time as possible.
- Records should be accurate and recorded in such a way that the meaning is clear.
- Records should be factual and not include unnecessary abbreviations, jargon, meaningless phrases or irrelevant speculation.
- Professional judgement should be used to decide what is relevant and what should be recorded.
- Details of any assessments and reviews undertaken should be included, and clear evidence provided of the arrangements you have made for future and ongoing care. This should also include details of information given about care and treatment.
- No records may be altered or destroyed without authorisation.
- Any alteration to your own or another healthcare professional's records must include your name and job title, and you should sign and date the original documentation. You should make sure that the alterations you make, and the original record, are clear and auditable.
- Where appropriate, the person in your care, or their carer, should be involved in the record-keeping process.
- Records should be readable when photocopied or scanned.
- You should not use coded expressions of sarcasm or humorous abbreviations to describe the people in your care.

ACTIVITY 3.3

Read Chapter 11 (Record keeping) in the following book:

Griffith, R. and Tengnah, C. (2017) *Law and Professional Issues in Nursing*, 4ᵗʰ edition (*Transforming Nursing Practice Series*). London: SAGE.

>> And finally...

Listed below are some of the common reasons why registered nurses are removed from the NMC register. Removal from the register is a result of the findings of Fitness to Practise panels where registered nurses' conduct and performance are measured against the *Code* (NMC, 2018a). Anyone has the right to complain to the NMC about a registered nurse – fellow registered nurses, colleagues in other healthcare professions, patients and their families, employers, managers and the police.

In October 2017 there were 287100 full-time equivalent nurses and health visitors working in hospitals and community health services in NHS England; in 2016–2017:
- 322 nurses were struck off the NMC register
- 384 were suspended
- 246 had condition of practice orders
- 153 had cautions.

Grounds for removal included:
- behaviour or violence
- communication issues
- criminal proceedings
- dishonesty
- employment and contractual issues
- information access
- investigations by other bodies
- management issues
- motor vehicle related
- NMC registration and proceedings
- not maintaining professional boundaries
- patient care
- prescribing and medicines management
- record-keeping
- registrant's health
- sexual offences
- other crimes and offences.

ACTIVITY 3.4

Obtain a copy of the *Code* (NMC, 2018a) from the NMC website (www.nmc.org.uk). Read it and then read the following article and identify the sections of the *Code* you think this nurse breached – the answers are in the conclusion at the end of the activity.

(Reproduced with permission from *British Journal of Nursing*)

ACTIVITY 3.4 (continued)

Staff nurse who failed to provide adequate nursing care for patients

British Journal of Nursing, 2004, Vol. 13, No 7:389 Professional Misconduct Series

In the following case a senior nurse called Jo deliberately ignored certain aspects of care while on night duty because she felt that it was not her responsibility to carry out certain tasks or to check that they had been done.

Jo worked on nights for a large inner-city hospital Trust and had been doing so for over 10 years. When working on the general medical/surgical wards she was often heard to say derogatory remarks about some of the patients or core nursing tasks she was expected to do. For example, she saw it as a junior nursing role to go round and attend to patients' pressure needs. She felt her expertise lay in giving out drugs, managing intravenous infusion lines and doing certain nursing procedures.

On the particular ward where she was working, two patients requested pain relief. Jo did not bother to go and see the patients, but instructed two healthcare assistants who were on duty with her to give each of the patients two paracetamol tablets. The healthcare assistants gave the medication to the patients as directed, but at no time did Jo attempt to check what they had been given or to clarify with the patients how they were feeling. The situation continued for several shifts. Any patient who required additional pain relief was referred by the healthcare assistants to Jo, who told them to give paracetamol.

On the last occasion that Jo and the healthcare assistants were on duty together, an agency nurse was also present because of the workload on the ward. However, Jo still did not help unless she felt it was absolutely necessary. At one time during the evening she left the ward for a break, stating that she had left the keys on the shelf in the office. These keys included keys to the controlled drug cupboard and the drugs trolley. Although Jo was entitled to a break from the ward, this was the third she had taken that night and she did not tell the staff where she was going.

The agency nurse was angry that Jo had left the ward without informing her of where she was going and how she could be contacted. Jo also did not tell the agency nurse where she could find the keys. A patient then complained of pain and the healthcare assistant asked the agency nurse, who was a registered nurse, if she could give the patient some paracetamol. The agency nurse then questioned the healthcare assistants about the procedure they had been following with Jo.

When Jo eventually returned to the ward, the agency nurse challenged her about the drug administration and leaving the keys in the ward office. Jo was offhand with the agency nurse and did not speak to her for the rest of the shift. At the handover to the day staff, Jo gave the report without involving the rest of the

ACTIVITY 3.4 (continued)

night nursing team. She let the healthcare assistants and the agency nurse write up the nursing records, but at no time in the handover did she involve them in the verbal report.

The agency nurse complained to the ward manager about the incidents that had occurred, and also some problems relating to a blood transfusion that Jo had been managing. It appeared that Jo had not followed the Trust protocol with regard to administration of a transfusion. There had been a long delay before it had been commenced and Jo had not recorded any observations of the patient during the transfusion.

Conclusion

An investigation was carried out by the Trust and it was felt that Jo should be dismissed from her post and her case referred to the Nursing and Midwifery Council. Jo was found guilty by the NMC of:

- failing to provide adequate support for patients on a ward
- giving medication to healthcare assistants to administer to patients
- leaving a ward without advising staff of her whereabouts, and not handing over the ward keys to a registered nurse colleague
- failing to provide an adequate and appropriate handover of patient care
- failing to follow the correct protocol and procedure while administering a blood transfusion.

The outcome was that Jo was removed from the nursing register.

Note: this case is part of a series based on true cases which were reported to the NMC.

CHAPTER SUMMARY

- Registered nurses are accountable in the criminal courts, the civil courts, before their employer and before the Fitness to Practise Committees of the NMC.
- Student nurses are similarly responsible to the criminal courts, civil courts, their university and placement provider and must act within *The Code: professional standards of practice and behaviour for nurses, midwives and nursing associates* (NMC, 2018a).
- Department of Health and NMC guidance for gaining consent, ensuring confidentiality and record-keeping must be adhered to.
- Government legislation and law need to be abided by and nurses have a responsibility to keep up to date.

Further information

This section has given a very brief introduction to the law. Further detail can be found in a variety of texts written for nurses, such as: Dimond's (2015) *Legal Aspects of Nursing*, 7ᵗʰ edition, and Griffith and Tengnah's (2017) *Law and Professional Issues in Nursing* (see reference list for further details). All Acts of Parliament can be found at: www.legislation.gov.uk

There is more detail on the role of the Nursing and Midwifery Council at: www.nmc.org.uk/about-us/our-role/

References

Berwick, D. (2013) *A Promise to Learn – A Commitment to Act: improving the safety of patients in England*. London: Department of Health.

Care Quality Commission (CQC) (2018) *Regulation 13: Safeguarding service users from abuse and improper treatment*. Available at: https://www.cqc.org.uk/guidance-providers/regulations-enforcement/regulation-13-safeguarding-service-users-abuse-improper (accessed 2 May 2019)

Caulfield, H. (2005) *Vital Notes for Nurses: accountability*. Oxford: Blackwell.

Department of Health (2009) *Reference Guide to Consent for Examination or Treatment* (2ⁿᵈ edition). London: DH.

Department of Health (2016) *Compassion in Practice: two years on*. Available at: www.england.nhs.uk/wp-content/uploads/2016/05/cip-two-years-on.pdf (accessed 4 April 2019)

Dimond, B. (2015) *Legal Aspects of Nursing* (7ᵗʰ edition). London: Pearson.

European Parliament (2016) *General Data Protection Regulation*. Available at: www.eugdpr.org/ (accessed 5 April 2019)

Francis, R. (2013) *Report of the Mid Staffordshire NHS Foundation Trust Public Inquiry*. London: The Stationery Office.

Griffith, R. and Tengnah, C. (2017) *Law and Professional Issues in Nursing*, 4ᵗʰ edition (*Transforming Nursing Practice Series*). London: SAGE.

Health Act (2006) Available at: www.legislation.gov.uk/ukpga/2006/28/contents (accessed 5 April 2019)

Keogh, B. (2013) *Review into the Quality of Care and Treatment Provided by 14 Hospital Trusts in England: overview report*. London: NHS England.

Mental Capacity Act (2007) Available at: www.legislation.gov.uk/uksi/2007/1897/contents/made (accessed 5 April 2019)

NHS Improvement (NHSI) (2016) *Freedom to Speak up: whistleblowing policy for the NHS*. Available at: https://improvement.nhs.uk/resources/freedom-to-speak-up-whistleblowing-policy-for-the-nhs/ (accessed 2 May 2019)

NHS Improvement (NHSI) (2018) *Better Healthcare, Transformed Care Delivery and Sustainable Finances*. Available from https://improvement.nhs.uk/ (accessed 2 May 2019)

Nursing and Midwifery (Amendment) Order (2016) Available at: www.gov.uk/government/uploads/system/uploads/attachment_data/file/518000/Nursing_and_Midwifery_Amendment_Order_2016_Draft_A.pdf (accessed 5 April 2019)

Nursing and Midwifery Council (2015a) *Openness and Honesty When Things go Wrong: the professional duty of candour*. Available at: https://www.nmc.org.uk/globalassets/sitedocuments/nmc-publications/openness-and-honesty-professional-duty-of-candour.pdf (accessed 5 April 2019)

Nursing and Midwifery Council (2018a) *The Code: professional standards of practice and behaviour for nurses, midwives and nursing associates*. London: NMC.

Nursing and Midwifery Council (2018b) *Future Nurse: standards of proficiency for registered nurses*. London: NMC.

Nursing and Midwifery Council (2019) *Guidance on Health and Character*. London: NMC. Available at: www.nmc.org.uk/globalassets/sitedocuments/registration/guidance-on-health-and-character.pdf (accessed 2 May 2019)

Peate, I. (2012) *The Student's Guide to Becoming a Nurse*, 2nd edition. Chichester: Wiley-Blackwell.

Peate, I. (2016) *The Essential Guide to Becoming a Staff Nurse*. Chichester: John Wiley & Sons Ltd.

Tingle, J. and Cribb, A. (eds) (2013) *Nursing Law and Ethics*, 4th edition. Chichester: John Wiley & Sons Ltd.

UK Caldicott Guardian Council (2017) *A Manual for Caldicott Guardians*. Available at: www.gov.uk/government/uploads/system/uploads/attachment_data/file/581213/cgmanual.pdf (accessed 5 April 2019)

VALUES AND HEALTHCARE ETHICS

The aim of this chapter is to outline some of the theories and principles used in the healthcare ethics and values debate.

As you work through this chapter, remember that no amount of reading will equip you with a set of absolute rules to solve all the moral problems you encounter. Tschudin (2003) believes ethics can only be described in terms of principles and never in terms of absolutes, while Aristotle is reputed to have said that 'there is a solution to every problem – the only problem is finding it!'

» Values and rights

"Values are different from factual knowledge because they are harder to quantify, standardise or provide evidence of; however, their impact on the care relationship is fundamental. Put simply, values are particular kinds of beliefs that are concerned with the worth or value of an idea or behaviour and are important in guiding our actions, our judgements, our behaviour and our attitudes towards others. In this way, values play an essential role in articulating the standards for the delivery of care and the manner in which the practitioner interacts with others in the care relationship."

(Cuthbert and Quallington, 2017, p. 5)

Chapter 3 included a discussion of the professional values, the 6Cs, which underpin our daily clinical practice. The term 'values' is often linked with the term 'ethics', which, in turn, is often used with the term 'morals'. According to Beauchamp and Childress (2013) morality refers to social conventions about right and wrong human conduct, whereas ethics is a general term referring to both morality and ethical theory. The NMC *Code* (NMC, 2018a) presents the professional values for nursing and aims to ensure that nurses act in

>> We are all influenced by our value system.

such a way to meet the needs of their patients that promotes and protects their interests (Walsh, 2018).

Your personal beliefs are the values that influence how you act (decision-making) and how you judge the actions of other people. Development of your personal moral 'knowledge' and values comes from a variety of sources: your upbringing and the personal values of your parents, gender, class, age, religious/spiritual beliefs, peer groups, culture, education, life experiences – the list could be endless. However, the important factor is that all your values are personal to you and frequently change as you progress through life, often through personal reflection (Walsh, 2018).

Every one of us is influenced by our value system. Values have the potential to motivate and guide our choices and decision-making abilities (Peate and Wild, 2018), but personal and professional values may not always be the same. Your values may also differ from those of another nurse, even though you are caring for the same patients. This is because they are personal and have been influenced by our families, culture, education, society, media, religious beliefs and our own individual experiences. Cuthbert and Quallington (2017) give the example of two healthcare workers working on a maternity ward who have very different views on abortion, but who are required to deliver the same professional care.

According to Hope (2004) most of us have 'gut reactions' as to what we think is morally right or wrong in certain situations. However, there are some viewpoints that most of us take into account when evaluating others' actions and behaviour, particularly in professional circumstances and regardless of our personal opinions:

- **Legal** – actions are right if they comply with the law, and wrong if they do not (see also *Chapter 3*).
- **Professional** – actions are right if they are supported by codes of professional conduct, protocols and evidence-based practice, and wrong if they are not.
- **Religious beliefs** – how does God or religious teaching view the action?
- **Social convention** – does the action conform to acceptable norms of behaviour in society?
- **Practical** – an action is right if it is the easiest and most practical way to achieve the desired aim or intention. Conflict will arise if it goes against any of the above or harms the patient.

Peate and Wild (2018) point out that nurses should remember that patients/ service users also have their own set of personal values, and this could lead to possible conflict. Fry and Johnstone (2008) therefore advise that nurses must respect the values of others, which is embedded in the NMC *Code* (NMC, 2018a), whilst ensuring that patients' rights are balanced with their own professional duties. NICE (2012) has also provided guidance on shared decision-making which places the patient/service user at the centre of their care.

» Patients' rights

Patients' rights are sometimes referred to as entitlements or claims and stem from the premise that individuals are unique and valuable and therefore should be afforded certain rights. These are sometimes described as 'positive rights' and 'negative rights'. Positive rights require society, or another individual, to do something positive in order to fulfil or uphold human and legal rights – for example, healthcare can only be realised if society ensures that healthcare systems exist and that the individuals in the system fulfil their duty to provide care. A negative right, sometimes referred to as a 'qualified right', relates to the freedom to do something without interference – for example, freedom of expression, or the freedom to practise one's preferred religion or not to practise a religion at all (Cuthbert and Quallington, 2017).

» Human rights

The major piece of international legislation relating to rights is the Human Rights Act (1998) (see also *Chapter 5*). This Act sets out what every person has a right to expect with regard to fundamental human rights and freedoms, regardless of gender, disability, ethnic identity, sexuality or class. It makes it unlawful for public authorities (and therefore nurses) to act in a way which is incompatible with the various articles within the Act.

> » **The Human Rights Act sets out what every person has a right to expect with regard to fundamental human rights and freedoms.**

Within the fourteen articles of the Human Rights Act, McHale and Gallagher (2004) differentiate between absolute rights, limited rights and qualified rights.

- **Absolute rights** cannot be restricted – for example, Article 2, 'The right to life' and Article 3, 'Prohibition of torture'.
- **Limited rights** include such articles as Article 5, 'Right to Liberty and Security', which contains a series of legitimate exceptions, such as "the lawful detention of persons for the prevention of the spreading of infectious diseases, of persons of unsound mind, alcoholics or drug addicts or vagrants".

- **Qualified rights** are found in Articles 8, 9 and 10 – 'Right to respect for private and family life', 'Freedom of thought, conscience and religion' and 'Freedom of expression', respectively – these fall into the same category as Cuthbert and Quallington's (2017) 'negative rights'.

The most pertinent of the fourteen articles to nursing are:
- **Article 8: Right to respect for private and family life, home and correspondence.** This confers the right for each person to live their own life as is reasonable within a democratic society, and takes account of the freedoms and rights of others. This right can also include the right to have personal information such as official records, including medical information, kept private and confidential. It also places restrictions on the extent to which any public authority can invade an individual's privacy about their body without their permission. In the healthcare context this has implications in relation to decisions of consent and refusal of treatment, and confidentiality of patient records. This Article provided the context and rationale for the former UK Data Protection Act (1998) which has recently been replaced with the UK General Data Protection Regulation (GDPR) (2018) (see also *Chapter 3*).
- **Article 9: Freedom of thought, conscience and religion.** This provides an absolute right for a person to hold the thoughts, positions of conscience or religion of their choice. This includes the right for the person to practise or demonstrate their religion in private or public (as long as it does not interfere with the rights and freedoms of others). In a healthcare setting this article is particularly applicable in relation to the right of healthcare professionals to opt out of certain procedures on the basis of conscientious objection; for example, assisting with pregnancy terminations. Equally it applies to patients who refuse treatment on religious grounds, such as Jehovah's Witnesses who may refuse transfusion of blood.
- **Article 14: Freedom from discrimination.** In the context of the Act discrimination is defined as "treating people in similar situations differently, or those in different situations in the same way, without proper justification" (Department for Constitutional Affairs, 2006, p. 25). Everyone is entitled to equal access to all the rights set out in the Act, regardless of personal status. Discrimination is prohibited on grounds of sex, sexual orientation, age, race, colour, language, religion, disability, political or other opinion, national or social origin, association with a national minority, property, birth (for example, whether a person is born inside or outside of marriage) and marital status (see also www.legislation.gov.uk).

These legal Articles provide the underpinning framework for the following UK Acts: Human Rights Act (1998), Equality Act (2010) and the Equality and Human Rights Act (2006) (Cuthbert and Quallington, 2017). In our multicultural society (see *Chapter 5*), these Acts legally bind nurses, and health and social care organisations, to embed anti-discriminatory practice in their daily work and so it is imperative that policies are in place and are followed in order to respect and value each individual and promote equality in all aspects of care, including access to services.

Breaches of these legal rights include criminal acts such as murder, manslaughter, rape and theft (all of which nurses have been found guilty of). The infringement of legal rights can also lead to civil cases, for example where an action for negligence results from a breach of duty of care (see also *Chapter 3*).

>> Professional considerations

Nurses must adhere to the NMC *Code* (NMC, 2018a) in order to maintain their registration. One of the primary functions of the NMC is to protect the public, and it publishes the standards of professional conduct that the public can expect of a registered practitioner (see www.nmc.org.uk). Any member of the public can access the NMC website and read the various standards and guidelines that indicate how they should be treated. In addition to the NMC *Code* there are various standards published by both the NMC and the Department of Health concerning issues such as confidentiality, consent, delivering competent care, advocacy and anti-discriminatory practice. They all outline patients' rights in these areas and emphasise the need for nurses to respect the standards. Other publications have statements about privacy, dignity and respect implicit within them – for example, National Service Frameworks, NICE (National Institute for Health and Care Excellence) guidelines, the Mental Capacity Act (2005), and so on.

The NHS Constitution (NHS England, 2015) establishes the principles and values of the NHS in England and sets out:

> "the rights to which patients, public and staff are entitled and pledges which the NHS is committed to achieve, together with responsibilities which the public, patients and staff owe to one another to ensure that the NHS operates fairly and effectively. The Secretary of State for Health, all NHS bodies, private and voluntary sector providers supplying NHS services, and local authorities in the exercise of their public health functions are required by law to take account of this Constitution in their decisions and actions."

(NHS England, 2015)

If you are based in a different region of the UK, the following principles and values information applies:
- Scotland: *Healthcare Principles* for Scotland (see www.nes.scot.nhs.uk/media/10978/Factsheet%201.pdf)

- Wales: *The Core Principles of NHS Wales* (see www.wales.nhs.uk/ nhswalesaboutus/thecoreprinciplesofnhswales)
- Northern Ireland: *Patient Standards* (see www.nidirect.gov.uk/articles/ patient-standards)

» Respect, dignity and privacy

The concepts of respect, dignity and privacy can be found in many healthcare professionals' codes of practice. Indeed, the first part of the NMC *Code* states that you must "treat people as individuals and uphold their dignity" (NMC, 2018a, Section 1) and "treat people with kindness, respect and compassion" (NMC 2018a, Clause 1.1). The words 'dignity' and 'respect' are often used together, in that dignity means being worthy of respect, and that giving a person respect will maintain their dignity. Cuthbert and Quallington (2017) believe nurses should respect everyone as a valued unique individual, and they cite Dillon (2014) as saying respect in care involves:

- a belief in the value of persons as individuals and as members of society
- treating people in the manner in which you would expect to be treated
- showing consideration for another person's feelings and interests
- an attitude demonstrating that you value another person.

Respect is shown in many ways, such as demonstrating a genuine interest in your patients, listening to them, preserving their modesty and addressing the patient by the name they prefer. However, there are other forms of respect that nurses have to acknowledge; 'respect for boundaries' such as the laws associated with consent, confidentiality, the professional relationship between a nurse and their patients, and within codes of conduct; and 'respect for authority' that you should show to personnel more senior to you.

Physical privacy can be hard to promote in a healthcare situation, and yet patients may be at their most vulnerable away from their familiar surroundings, and yearn for privacy. Many environments do not lend themselves to privacy – for example, mixed sex wards, bedpans behind curtains, personal hygiene needs and so on. However, treating the patient with dignity and respect at these times can go a long way to enhancing care where privacy may be compromised. Remember that privacy also extends to the patient's space and belongings. In their own environment this is relatively easy for people to control, but in a healthcare setting patients are often unable to limit the power of others to intrude.

Respect and dignity are part of the benchmarks published by the Department of Health (2010) in its document *Essence of Care*. This is a set of guidelines aimed at promoting good person-centred care organised around 'factors' and 'benchmarks'. The benchmarks for respect and dignity are shown in *Table 4.1*.

Table 4.1: *Benchmarks of* Essence of Care *(Department of Health, 2010, p. 262)*.

Factor	Benchmark
1. Attitudes and behaviours	Patients feel that they matter all of the time
2. Personal world and personal identity	Patients experience care in an environment that actively encompasses individual values, beliefs and personal relationships
3. Personal boundaries and space	Patients' personal space is actively promoted by all staff
4. Communicating with staff and patients	Communication between staff and patients takes place in a manner which respects their individuality
5. Privacy of patient and confidentiality of patient information	Patient information is shared to enable care, with their consent
6. Privacy, dignity and modesty	Patients' care actively promotes their privacy and dignity, and protects their modesty
7. Availability of an area for complete privacy	Patients and/or carers can access an area that safely provides privacy

Privacy = freedom from intrusion; *Dignity* = being worthy of respect

To ensure that these guidelines, and indeed all Department of Health guidelines and standards, are upheld, the government established the Care Quality Commission (CQC) in 2009. This body is the independent regulator of health and social care in England, and its aim is to make sure better care is provided for everyone, whether in hospitals, care homes, people's own homes or elsewhere. To that end it regulates health and adult social care services provided by the NHS, local authorities, private companies and voluntary organisations (see also *Chapter 6*).

RECAP

- Everyone is influenced by their value system, and that includes your patients and service users.
- Patient have rights that include the fundamental rights established under the Human Rights Act and those that are stipulated in professional and ethical codes, such as respect, dignity and privacy.

ACTIVITY 4.1

How would you ensure that "patients experience care in an environment that actively encompasses individual values, beliefs and personal relationships" (benchmark 2)? Make brief notes.

>> Healthcare ethics

The text in this section was adapted from the work of Dr Ian Donaldson of the Faculty of Health and Social Sciences, Bournemouth University.

The NMC (2018b, p. 8) states that a nurse needs to understand ethics and ethical frameworks. Burnard and Chapman (2003) note that the term 'ethics' is notoriously ambiguous, conjuring up different images for different people. It is important to recognise that every individual will have differing opinions and views, and sometimes there are no right or wrong attitudes or beliefs. As they also explain, ethics informs how we choose to act in a morally good and right way, both personally and professionally, and guides our decision-making. Everyone should be able to express their views, while remembering not to exclude alternative viewpoints, as ethical debate is about individuals reflecting on their own and others' viewpoints with insight and reasoning.

Nurses are often confronted with moral dilemmas – this is when they recognise that they both ought and ought not to perform a particular action as there are equally compelling reasons for and against it. This is made increasingly difficult when nurses have differing views and values, often causing disagreements between colleagues or with patients.

Griffith and Tengnah (2017) give the example of a nurse who believes a doctor's decision not to resuscitate a patient with a terminal illness is wrong – the nurse believes the patient's life should be sustained, and is suddenly faced with a dilemma about what is right or wrong. Both decisions are lawful, so the decision is one of morality. Another good example of this can be found in the constant debate about abortion – whose rights prevail?

Using theories and principles may help to guide moral deliberations. There are a wide range of differing moral standpoints but three particular ways of moral reasoning have been extremely influential in the shaping and discussions of healthcare ethics. They are the theories of utilitarianism and deontology, and the principles of healthcare ethics.

Utilitarianism

This idea was first put forward by Jeremy Bentham in the 18th century and refined by John Stuart Mill in the 19th century. Mill believed that the way to evaluate what was morally right or wrong was to examine the outcome or 'consequences' of that action – whether the action produces good consequences, and not just whether it was done with good intentions. Mill's golden rule was that actions are right if they promote happiness and wrong if they

>> Utilitarianism suggests that actions are right if they produce the greatest good to the greatest number.

produce the reverse of happiness. This rule is often abbreviated to 'the greatest happiness or the greatest good to the greatest number' and that 'the end (the consequences) justifies the means (the action taken)'.

An argument against utilitarianism is that it can promote activities that are a selfish pursuit of pleasure at the expense of everyone else. Mill attempted to solve this critique with two additional 'rules'. He said that actions were good if they created the greatest amount of happiness. This argument means that selfish activities that create happiness for one person but unhappiness in a great deal of other people are not acceptable (for example, consider how this 'rule' prevents a paedophile from justifying his actions). Mill's second 'rule' was that there is a difference between the quantity and quality of pleasures that cause happiness. He believes that it is better to pursue high quality pleasures, which he describes as intellectual, aesthetic and imaginative, rather than lower quality pleasures which he describes as 'mere animal instincts'.

A major criticism of utilitarianism is that one cannot predict consequences with certainty; utilitarianism is therefore not useful in guiding individuals as to what they ought to do. Included in the definition of utilitarianism is the 'rightness or wrongness of an action' and whether it furthers the goal of the greatest happiness for the greatest number (Thompson *et al.*, 2006).

This can have implications, for example in a common situation nurses face, which is telling the truth. As a nurse you would have to weigh up the consequences as to whether telling the truth would lead to more 'happiness' than 'unhappiness'. In this instance, it can be very difficult to evaluate the potential long-term benefit to the patient (of knowing the truth) versus the short-term distress (of learning bad news). It is for this reason that some prefer not to use a utilitarian approach, preferring instead to explore what is the right thing to do using a different theory. The theory of deontology is examined below.

Deontology

The theory of deontology was put forward by Kant in the 18th century. He believed it is the action that is important and not the consequences. Kant was also concerned with the motive and intentions of the individual performing the action, and argued that the action is only morally right if the individual is motivated by goodwill. Kant's theory is often called the dutiful view of morality, where we are bound by duty to act in a particular way, and not to produce certain consequences.

» Deontology holds that an action is right if it is motivated by goodwill.

You may consider that certain actions such as being honest, telling the truth and keeping a promise are right and good actions, but how can an individual decide where their duty lies? Kant argues that we know where our duty lies by considering this question: 'Do I want everyone to behave as I am proposing to do in these circumstances?' This he called the 'categorical imperative', or a universal law. An example of this could be to 'always keep a promise' because you would want others to keep their promises to you – this is therefore something that you would want to be a universal law.

Kant's theory of deontology is criticised for the problems it can create when a categorical imperative, such as always telling the truth, is followed in every situation. However, this criticism seems to miss the point on two counts – first, for many the idea that certain actions are right in themselves and ought to be followed is an important part of their view of morality; secondly, it ignores the process by which the truth is told.

It is important to stress that while both these theories of utilitarianism (concerned with the outcome) and deontology (concerned with the motive) are different, they do not always lead to different evaluations of a particular action (Peate and Wild, 2018).

Principles of healthcare ethics

Beauchamp and Childress wrote their very influential book in the late 1970s (various editions have been produced since), and many nurses refer to this text. They suggest that there are four key principles in healthcare ethics, and argue that by examining a dilemma using these principles the nurse will be helped to decide what the right course of action is. Therefore, these principles are not rules but can be used to guide morally right behaviour.

The key principles are:
- respect for Autonomy
- Beneficence
- Non-maleficence
- Justice.

Autonomy

Autonomy is defined as "the capacity to think, decide and act on the basis of such thought and decision ... freely and independently without let or hindrance" (Gillon, 1986, p. 6). Autonomy is seen as being increasingly important within healthcare, and is closely allied to respect for people's choices and individuality. It is also referred to as self-determination or self-rule (Peate and Wild, 2018).

Cuthbert and Quallington (2017, p. 121) suggest that definitions of autonomy often include references to such terms as:
- self-governance
- independence
- individuality
- self-choice/individual choice
- freedom/freedom of will
- being one's own person.

Autonomy is linked with many issues in nursing, including values, respect and privacy. In terms of values, Beauchamp and Childress (2013) suggest respect for autonomy is based on the general recognition that an individual has unconditional worth, with the capacity to determine their own destiny. Dworkin (1988) believes that people know what is best for them, so giving them the right to express their autonomy will contribute to their happiness and wellbeing.

Patients' autonomy can be compromised when they enter a healthcare setting. What were previously everyday decisions can be taken away from them and this is disempowering: for example, what to wear, when to shower, when and what to eat, where and when to sleep. Peate and Wild (2018) point out that talking with the patient and their family can ensure that the patient retains as much autonomous decision-making as possible, and this is a key aspect of the nurse's role. Thompson *et al.* (2006) further suggest that nurses should actually protect patients who suffer loss of autonomy through illness, injury or mental disorder.

Cuthbert and Quallington (2017, p. 142) state that respecting autonomy is not "about agreeing with the wishes of others" but is about nurses and other healthcare professionals enabling and empowering patients/service users to express their personal preferences and make their own reasoned decisions. This involves using effective communication skills (see also *Chapter 2*) to provide the required information in an appropriate and meaningful way to the individual in a supportive environment (Cuthbert and Quallington, 2017).

The NMC *Code* (2018a) upholds the patient's right to autonomy in many ways; it advocates confidentiality, consent, privacy and dignity, among other important issues concerned with autonomy. Dworkin (1988) considers these (particularly consent) and states that the patient's autonomy depends on certain conditions:

- the ability to make independent choices
- adequate information
- adequate knowledge.

For example, it is well recognised in the UK that any mentally competent adult has the right in law to consent to any touching of his or her person (the law relating to children giving consent is different). For an individual to give consent, and so exercise their autonomy, it is clear that information is required to enable an informed decision to be made; for example, when taking a blood pressure. Equally, adults have the right to refuse treatment and as nurses we need to accept and respect their decisions. The Montgomery Consent Rule has enshrined informed consent as a legal requirement and having the capacity to consent is discussed in *Chapter 3* (RCN, 2017).

Paternalism

When an individual acts to override someone's autonomy by restricting information or choices, it is described as paternalism. This is done with the intention of benefiting that person, but it takes away their choice (for example, a doctor advocating surgery when the patient does not want an operation). It is always very difficult to know the right course of action in this type of situation.

A guide could be to remember that respect for autonomy is of central importance when considering a patient's request, and to ask yourself two questions. First, is the patient mentally competent or is there a situation where a patient's capacity to make an informed decision will compromise their autonomy? (see *Chapter 3*). Secondly, does the consideration rest on whether one of the other principles (beneficence, non-maleficence or justice) carries greater weight in the particular situation?

It is also useful to refer to the NMC *Code* (2018a) which outlines the nurse's role in gaining consent.

Beneficence

Beneficence is the duty to do good and avoid doing harm to others (both physically and psychologically), and has been described as "do unto others as you would have them do unto you" (Thompson *et al.*, 2006). As a nurse you have a duty of care to your patients (NMC, 2018a) and a duty to promote what is best for your patients. This has been the guiding principle in healthcare for some time, and is accomplished by acting in the patient's 'best interests'.

However, acting in the patient's best interests raises the question of who should be the judge of what is best for the patient (Hope, 2004). Linked with the principle of autonomy, it should be the patient who decides, but in some instances this is not possible. The Mental Capacity Act (2005) recognises this and is concerned with protecting those who lack the capacity to make their own decisions or consent to treatment in a variety of health and social care circumstances – this can either be on a temporary or permanent basis (see *Chapter 3*).

The principle of beneficence can cause tensions if a competent patient decides on an action which is not in their best interests – for example, a Jehovah's Witness refusing a life-saving blood transfusion. If action was taken, the hospital staff would be "violating the bodily integrity of the person without consent" (Hope, 2004), which in legal terms would amount to committing battery.

Seedhouse (2009) includes truth-telling in his discussion of beneficence, and believes it is a central principle of conduct. However, he also believes there are some instances when it is better not to tell the truth, thereby propounding the principle of non-maleficence. He gives the example of allowing patients to read their medical records. Truth-telling relates closely to respect for the person and their autonomy, particularly when it comes to giving information on which people will base their choices and decisions in health and care (Cuthbert and Quallington, 2017). Indeed the NMC (2018a) states that nurses should communicate with people in their care in terms they can understand.

ACTIVITY 4.2

Consider a situation from your placements when information was withheld.
- Was this justified?
- What ethical, legal and professional implications arose from this type of action?
- How was the situation resolved?
- Do you think this was satisfactory? If not, why not?

Non-maleficence

This principle states 'above all to do no harm'. Although many nursing interventions may cause harm in order to successfully treat a patient – for example, chemotherapy – it is clear that to intentionally cause distress is morally wrong. Beauchamp and Childress (2013) point out that obligations not to harm are sometimes more stringent than obligations to help. The NMC *Code* (2018a, p. 13) states that you must ensure that patient and public safety is protected and raise your concerns when you encounter situations that put the patient or public at risk. Apart from the ethical aspects of this, failure to comply could bring a court action for negligence.

ACTIVITY 4.3

Can you think of a situation where harm could be caused to a patient, but in the long term it would be in their best interests? How do you feel about this situation?

Justice

The final principle to consider is that of justice where "everyone is valued equally and treated alike" (Peate and Wild, 2012, p. 98). According to Hope (2004, p. 66) there are four elements to this principle:

- **Distributive justice** (sometimes termed entitlement): patients in similar situations should normally have access to the same healthcare and, in determining what level of healthcare should be available for one set of patients, account should be taken of the effect of such a use of resources on other patients. In other words, limited resources should be distributed fairly.
- **Respect for the law:** the fact that an act is, or is not, within the law is of moral relevance. Some people may take the view that it might in some situations be morally right to break the law, but laws are made through a democratic process and have to be enforced.
- **Rights:** the fundamental idea that a person has rights is a safeguard to their rights being respected, even if overall the social good is thereby diminished.
- **Retributive justice:** concerns the fitting of punishment to the crime – an element not really concerned with healthcare provision.

When considering distributive justice or 'entitlement', there is a range of different options for the allocation of resources in healthcare:
- equal share to everyone
- random distribution
- on a first come, first served basis
- according to need
- to deserving cases
- to treat as many as possible.

Some of these options can in themselves create inequalities. For example, to allocate an equal share of a resource to everyone may in some cases be perceived as wrong, because some individuals are disadvantaged as they have a greater need.

CHAPTER SUMMARY

- The words values, ethics and morals are often used interchangeably.
- Different viewpoints shape individuals' behaviour towards each other.
- Everyone has fundamental rights under the Human Rights Act.
- Respect, dignity and privacy are key concepts when delivering nursing care.
- Principles of healthcare ethics should be considered when caring for patients.

Further information

Values and Ethics for Care Practice by Sue Cuthbert and Jan Quallington (Lantern Publishing, 2017) provides a detailed exploration of healthcare values.

References

Beauchamp, T. and Childress, J. (2013) *Principles of Biomedical Ethics*, 7th edition. Oxford: Oxford University Press.

Burnard, P. and Chapman, C. (2003) *Professional and Ethical Issues in Nursing*, 3rd edition. London: Baillière Tindall.

Cuthbert, S. and Quallington, J. (2017) *Values and Ethics for Care Practice*. Banbury: Lantern Publishing Ltd.

Department for Constitutional Affairs (2006) *A Guide to the Human Rights Act 1998*, 3rd edition. London: DCA.

Department of Health (2005) *The Mental Capacity Act*. London: HMSO.

Department of Health (2010) *Essence of Care: benchmarks for the fundamental aspects of care*. London: DH.

Dillon, R. (2014) *Respect, The Stanford Encyclopedia of Philosophy* (Spring 2014 edition), Edward N. Zalta (ed.). Available at https://plato.stanford.edu/archives/spr2014/entries/respect/ (accessed 5 April 2019), in: Cuthbert, S. and Quallington, J. (2017) *Values and Ethics for Care Practice*. Banbury: Lantern Publishing Ltd.

Dworkin, G. (1988) *The Theory and Practice of Autonomy*. Cambridge: Cambridge University Press.

Fry, S. and Johnstone, M-J. (2008) *Ethics in Nursing Practice: a guide to ethical decision making*, 3rd edition. Chichester: Wiley-Blackwell.

Gillon, R. (1986) *Philosophical Medical Ethics*. Chichester: Wiley.

Griffith, R. and Tengnah, C. (2017) *Law and Professional Issues in Nursing*, 4th edition (*Transforming Nursing Practice Series*). London: SAGE.

Hope, T. (2004) *Medical Ethics: a very short introduction*. Oxford: Oxford University Press.

McHale, J. and Gallagher, A. (2004) *Nursing and Human Rights*. Edinburgh: Butterworth-Heinemann.

NHS England (2015) *NHS Constitution for England*. Available at: www.gov.uk/government/publications/the-nhs-constitution-for-england (accessed 5 April 2019)

NICE (2012) *Shared Decision Making*. Available at: www.nice.org.uk/about/what-we-do/our-programmes/nice-guidance/nice-guidelines/shared-decision-making (accessed 5 April 2019)

Nursing and Midwifery Council (2018a) *The Code: professional standards of practice and behaviour for nurses, midwives and nursing associates*. London: NMC.

Nursing and Midwifery Council (2018b) *Future Nurse: standards of proficiency for registered nurses*. London: NMC.

Peate, I. and Wild, K. (2018) *Nursing Practice: knowledge and care*. Chichester: Wiley-Blackwell.

Royal College of Nursing (2017) *Principles of Consent Guidance for Nursing Staff.* London: RCN.

Seedhouse, D. (2009) *Ethics: the heart of health care*, 3rd edition. Chichester: Wiley.

Thompson, I., Melia, K., Boyd, K., and Horsburgh, D. (2006) *Nursing Ethics*, 5th edition. Edinburgh: Churchill Livingstone.

Tschudin, V. (2003) *Ethics in Nursing: the caring relationship*, 3rd edition. London: Butterworth-Heinemann.

Walsh, M. (2018) *Key Topics in Social Sciences: an A–Z guide for student nurses.* Banbury: Lantern Publishing Ltd.

Useful websites

https://www.gov.uk/guidance/equality-act-2010-guidance (accessed 5 April 2019)

www.legislation.gov.uk (accessed 5 April 2019)

www.nmc.org.uk (accessed 5 April 2019)

CULTURAL AWARENESS

The aim of this chapter is to explore briefly the concept of culture and to raise your awareness of cultural/religious considerations relating to the delivery of healthcare within a culturally diverse society.

LEARNING OUTCOMES

On completion of this chapter you should be able to:
- discuss the concept of culture and understand the associated terminology
- outline current legislation important to practice
- appraise the customs and factors that may have an impact on the provision, delivery and receipt of healthcare for some patients/service users
- reflect on your own personal experiences of the multicultural dimensions of care
- outline key issues associated with transcultural care that are needed to deliver non-discriminatory, culturally sensitive and person-centred care

>> Introduction

The population of the UK, like that of many European countries, has been shaped considerably by post-war patterns of emigration and immigration. The 2011 Census highlights the fact that there continues to be an increasing number of people identifying with minority ethnic groups in the UK. In England and Wales a total of seventeen different ethnic groups were recorded, representing approximately 19% of the overall population in these two regions (ONS, 2012). In Scotland, the census found that 4% of the total population identified themselves as ethnic, based on the classifications provided (Scottish Government, 2012) and in Northern Ireland it was 1.8% (Northern Ireland Assembly, 2013).

>> Nurses must provide and promote non-discriminatory, person-centred and sensitive care at all times.

It is therefore easy to understand why the UK is now considered to be a multicultural, multi-ethnic and multifaith society. As a nurse you are required to make "accurate, culturally aware assessments of care needs" and ensure that "the needs, priorities, expertise and preferences of people are always valued and taken into account" (NMC, 2018a, p. 27). This requires the nurse to "provide and promote non-discriminatory, person-centred and sensitive care at all times, reflecting on people's values and beliefs, diverse backgrounds, cultural characteristics, language requirements, needs and preferences, taking account of any need for adjustments" (NMC, 2018a, p. 9). This includes the care provided for a deceased person and the bereaved where it is necessary to respect "cultural requirements and protocols" (NMC, 2018a, p. 36).

This chapter explores the concept of culture, the relevant legislation and policy (see also *Chapter 4*) and religious awareness.

» Culture

According to Walsh (2018), culture is a concept that is multifaceted, engenders much discussion and suggests the notion of a group of people bound together collectively. Papadopoulos (2006, p. 13) explains that culture "is the shared way of life of a group of people that includes beliefs, values, ideas, language, communication, norms and visibly expressed forms such as customs, art, music, clothing and etiquette. Culture influences individuals' lifestyles, personal identity and their relationship with others both within and outside their culture". A review of the literature – for example, Papadopoulous (2006), Andrews and Boyle (2015) and Jirwe (2008) – identifies four main characteristics of culture:

1. It is **learned** from birth through the process of language acquisition and socialisation. From society's point of view, socialisation is the way culture is transmitted and the individual is fitted into the group's organised way of life.
2. It is **shared** by all members of the same cultural group; in fact it is the sharing of cultural beliefs and patterns that binds people together under one identity as a group (even though this is not always a conscious process).
3. It is an **adaptation** to specific activities related to environmental and technical factors and to the availability of natural resources.
4. It is a **dynamic**, ever-changing process. People do not merely receive their culture from others, they also make it and remake it continually in a process of interaction with others.

Hofstede *et al.* (2010) also identify numerous layers of culture which include:

• national
• regional
• gender

- generational
- professional
- organisational
- social class.

Finally, Giger (2017) suggests that the following cultural phenomena exist:
- **Communication** – there is no known culture without a grammatically complex language, with different languages having different meanings.
- **Social organisation** – family systems and religious and other organisation groups vary among cultures.
- **Space** – various cultures have different concepts about social and personal space and territory.
- **Time** – each culture has its own conception and orientation of time.
- **Environmental control** – the values, beliefs and concepts of health practices vary widely among cultural groups. If it is not easy to understand the logic of a particular belief or practice, that does not mean there is no logic behind it; it need not be logically based on the laws of western society and medical science to be valid and practical.
- **Biological considerations** – constitutional endowment and vulnerability differ among people representing different cultures.

>> Associated cultural terminology

Terminology closely associated with the term 'culture' includes the terms ethnicity, ethnocentrism and race.

Ethnicity

There does not appear to be a single, universally accepted concept of ethnicity and this in itself can pose challenges for nurses caring for patients from multi-ethnic groups. It is generally perceived as a term that represents a given social group with a shared history, sense of identity, country of origin, language, religion and cultural practices that characterise and distinguish them from other groups (Walsh, 2018).

Ethnocentrism

According to Macionis and Plummer (2011) this term refers to "the practice of judging another culture by the standards of one's own culture" and it can imply the assumption that one's own cultural group is superior to that of others. Clearly, to adopt such an approach would be totally against providing non-discriminatory and holistic care to individual patients.

Race

Klein (1971) suggests the word 'race' may have initially meant 'to unite' or 'to join'. Later it was used more loosely for national groups such as, for example, the French or German race. In the 19th century, scientists took it over to describe the 'races of man'; groups defined by their physical appearance from one another, in aspects such as skin colour, hair type and body shape, etc. Numerous theories were developed about these different races, which have now long since been discredited as unscientific and wrong. Race is now widely acknowledged as a social/political construct rather than a biological or genetic fact.

Within the definition of culture and its associated terms it is important to remember that it includes historical, present and future dimensions and has immense implications for the nursing care you need to provide. Culture is not homogenous and therefore generalisations about individual members from a group should not be made, as they can lead to stereotypical attitudes, cultural misunderstanding, prejudices and discrimination (Jirwe, 2008).

>> Legislation and policy

As a nurse there are two main pieces of legislation relating to cultural diversity that you need to be familiar with.

The Human Rights Act (1998)

The Human Rights Act came into force in October 2000. It represents the translation of the law of the European Convention on Human Rights into the laws of the UK. This means that the UK has a legislative framework that defines standards for what each person has a right to expect with regard to fundamental human rights and freedoms. The Act covers all infringements of human rights regardless of gender, disability, ethnic identity, sexuality or class and makes it unlawful for public authorities (which includes NHS Trusts, all health authorities, private and voluntary sector contractors, social services, general practitioners, dentists, opticians and pharmacists) to act in a way that is incompatible with Convention rights, unless they are acting under legislation which makes it impossible to act differently. The Convention rights include the following:

- **Article 2: The right to life** – The state is required to make adequate provision in its laws for the protection of human life. This means it must take positive steps to protect life in all kinds of situations, including admission to hospital and other healthcare settings. Hospitals are under a duty to take positive steps to safeguard a patient's right to life. Relevant healthcare staff may therefore need to consider the implications before refusing life-saving treatment to a patient.

- **Article 3: Freedom from torture and inhuman or degrading treatment or punishment** – This is an absolute right not to be tortured or subjected to treatment or punishment that is inhuman or degrading. How an individual's treatment is classified depends on many different factors, including their state of health. Whether or not treatment is considered degrading depends on "whether a reasonable person of the same age or sex and health as you would have felt degraded" (DCA, 2006, p. 16).
- **Article 4: Freedom from slavery and forced or compulsory labour** – This is an absolute right not be treated like a slave or forced to perform certain kinds of labour. This might apply to a situation such as staff from overseas having their passports removed by their employers to prevent them leaving a place of work.
- **Article 5: Right to liberty, freedom and security of person** – Unless a detention is lawful, an individual cannot be deprived of their liberty for even a short period of time. Detention in this context can include detention in mental hospitals. Acceptable reasons for arrest and detention, in accordance with set procedures set down by law, include: "if a person is shown to be of unsound mind, an alcoholic, a drug addict or a vagrant", or to prevent an individual spreading infectious disease.
- **Article 6: Right to a fair trial** – Every person has the right to a fair hearing, a public hearing, an independent and impartial tribunal and to a hearing within a reasonable time.
- **Article 7: Freedom from retrospective criminal law and no punishment without law** – This relates to the right to normally not be found guilty of a criminal offence that occurred at a time when the offence was not deemed a criminal act.
- **Article 8: Right to respect for private and family life, home and correspondence** – This confers the right for each person to live their own life as is reasonable within a democratic society and takes account of the freedoms and rights of others. This right can also include the right to have personal information such as official records, including medical information, kept private and confidential. This right also places restrictions on the extent to which any public authority can invade an individual's privacy about their body without their permission. It should be noted that this raises issues in procedures such as taking blood samples and the right to refuse treatment.
- **Article 9: Freedom of thought, conscience and religion** – This provides an absolute right for a person to hold the thoughts, positions of conscience or religion of their choice. This includes the right for the person to practise or demonstrate their religion in private or public (as long as it does not interfere with the rights and freedoms of others).
- **Article 10: Freedom of expression** – 'Expression' here includes personal views or opinions, speaking aloud, publication of articles or books or leaflets, television

or radio broadcasting, producing works of art, communication through the internet, and some forms of commercial information (DCA, 2006, p. 23).

- **Article 11: Freedom of assembly and association** – Every person has the right to 'peacefully' assemble with others.
- **Article 12: Right to marry** – This includes the right to have a family.
- **Article 14: Freedom from discrimination** – In the context of the Act, discrimination is defined as "treating people in similar situations differently, or those in different situations in the same way, without proper justification" (DCA, 2006, p. 25). Among other issues this includes sexual orientation, age, race, colour, language, religion, disability, political or other opinion, national or social origin, association with a national minority, property, birth (for example whether born inside or outside of marriage), and marital status.

Regardless of status, everyone is entitled to equal access to all the rights set out in the Act.

- **Protocol 1 of Article 2: Right to education** – No person should be denied the right to the education system and an effective education.

Articles 2, 3, 8, 9 and 14 are particularly important to nursing practice and relate to the Nursing and Midwifery Council *Code* (2018b, Clause 1.5).

ACTIVITY 5.1

Research further information regarding the Human Rights Act 1998 from www.direct.gov.uk, www.YourRights.org.uk, www.dh.gov.uk, www.bihr.org.uk or through a general search engine such as Google. Then consider and note down the implications of Articles 2, 3, 8, 9 and 14 in relation to your practice as a student of nursing and the NMC (2018b) *Code: professional standards of practice and behaviour for nurses, midwives and nursing associates.*

The Equality Act 2010

The Equality Act 2010 is the law that seeks to ban unfair treatment and achieve equal opportunities in the workplace and wider society. It brought together nine pieces of previous legislation under one Act with an aim to provide a fairer and more equal society (Equality and Human Rights Commission, 2017).

The Act covers nine 'protected characteristics':
- age
- race
- religion or belief
- disability

- gender identity and gender reassignment
- sex
- sexual orientation
- pregnancy and maternity
- marriage and civil partnership.

The Equality Act sets out the different ways in which it is unlawful to treat someone, for example by direct or indirect discrimination, harassment or victimisation, and failing to make a reasonable adjustment for a disabled person (Equality and Human Rights Commission, 2017).

It covers all aspects of an organisation's activities, policy and service provision and delivery, as well as employment practices. This obviously has considerable implications for your work, both as a student nurse and a registered nurse.

RECAP

- The NMC requires nurses to provide non-discriminatory care to everyone regardless of their cultural and ethnic background.
- The two key pieces of legislation that nurses need to be familiar with in relation to non-discrimination are the Human Rights Act and the Equality Act.

ACTIVITY 5.2

Referring to the Equality Act (2010) (see www.gov.uk/guidance/equality-act-2010-guidance) consider and note down the implications of this Act in relation to your practice as a nursing student and the NMC (2018b) *Code: professional standards of practice and behaviour for nurses, midwives and nursing associates.* London: NMC.

>> Culture in practice

As already noted, given the population profile of the UK, you will care for patients from a variety of cultural, religious and ethnic backgrounds, which will require you to have an understanding of the knowledge and skills required for effective transcultural nursing.

McFarland and Wehbe-Alamah (2018) suggest that transcultural nursing is theory and practice that focuses specifically on comparing the care for people with differences and similarities in beliefs, values and cultures in order to provide meaningful and beneficial healthcare. The 6Cs (Department of

Health and NHS Commissioning Board, 2012) are values which underpin anti-discriminatory and compassionate care for all. More specific models have been developed such as Narayanasamy's (2002) transcultural nursing practice framework, ACCESS, which is one practical approach:

- **Assessment**: Focus on cultural aspects of client's lifestyle, health beliefs, and health practices.
- **Communication**: Be aware of variations in verbal and non-verbal responses.
- **Cultural negotiation and compromise**: Become more aware of aspects of other people's culture as well as understanding clients' views and explaining their problems.
- **Establishing respect and rapport**: A therapeutic relation is required which portrays genuine respect for clients' cultural beliefs and values.
- **Sensitivity**: Deliver culturally sensitive care to a culturally diverse group.
- **Safety**: Enable clients to derive a sense of cultural safety.

(Narayanasamy, 2002, p. 645)

Papadopoulos *et al.* (cited by Papadopoulous, 2006), set out a model for developing cultural competency in care delivery. Their model comprises four stages:

1. **Self-awareness**, which requires us to understand our own individual values and beliefs (see also *Chapter 4*).
2. **Cultural Knowledge**, which requires exploration and understanding of health beliefs and behaviours, bio-psycho-social understanding as well as similarities and differences between cultures and health inequalities.
3. The third stage is **Cultural Sensitivity** which includes "empathy, interpersonal/ communication skills [see also *Chapter 2*], trust and respect, acceptance, appropriateness [of actions and behaviours] [and being aware of the potential] barriers to cultural sensitivity" (ibid., p. 10) such as non-verbal communication, clock time, use of names (ibid., p. 18).
4. The fourth aspect is **Cultural Competence**, with a focus on "assessment skills, diagnostic skills, clinical skills [and] challenging and addressing prejudice, discrimination and inequalities" (ibid., p. 10).

Each stage links to the next and the fourth stage links back to the first stage, Self-awareness.

Therefore, as well as learning and understanding the cultural values, behavioural patterns and interaction in specific cultures, it is necessary for you to explore your personal values, beliefs and attitudes and the professional values associated with nursing. This enables you to develop the skills and knowledge to be culturally competent and deliver person-centred, culturally sensitive care which will improve not only the safety and quality of patient care but also their health outcomes.

ACTIVITY 5.3

Reflect and note down your cultural values, beliefs and attitudes and consider how important they are to you.

The NMC *Code* (2018b, Clause 7.3) identifies that delivering non-discriminatory and culturally sensitive person-centred care will require you to "use a range of verbal and non-verbal communication methods, and consider cultural sensitivities, to better understand and respond to people's personal and health needs" (see also *Chapter 2*). In addition, it states that you must "avoid making assumptions and recognise diversity and individual choice" (NMC, 2018b, Clause 1.3). Furthermore, you are required to be able to "provide care for the deceased person and the bereaved, respecting cultural requirements and protocols" (NMC, 2018a, p. 36).

» Religious awareness

In order to deliver care that is non-discriminatory, culturally sensitive and individual, nurses should seek to ensure that they deliver holistic care that respects the religious, spiritual, dietary and linguistic requirements of patients, as well as encompassing the values and beliefs of their wider family/carers.

The following brief notes seek to remind you, or raise your awareness of, some differing religious beliefs you may encounter while working as a nurse.

Christianity

Christians believe in the Holy Trinity of one God, the father of mankind who created heaven and earth, and who sent his son Jesus Christ to save mankind, and then sent the Holy Spirit to continue his work in human affairs. Christians believe that everything is created and given life by God the Father. Christianity stresses the importance of living a good life in response to God's love. It encompasses many groups and sects, but the main ones in the UK are the Anglican Church (which includes the Church of England, Church of Wales, Church of Scotland and Church of Ireland), the Roman Catholic Church, the free or non-conformist churches (for example, the Baptist Church, Methodist Church) and the Eastern Orthodox Churches (for example the Greek and Russian Orthodox Churches).

The Christian holy book is the Bible, the interpretation of which can differ between sects or groups. Thus it has implications for delivery and acceptance of treatment and care. It is therefore very important that you establish from the outset to which Christian sect or group an individual may belong.

Considerations for practice

Diet

Most Christians do not follow religious dietary restrictions, although some may wish not to eat meat on Fridays, Ash Wednesday or Good Friday. They should therefore be offered a fish or vegetarian alternative.

Prayers

Some Christians may wish to receive Holy Communion and, possibly, the Anointing of the Sick, which involves being anointed with holy oil. A private and, where possible, quiet area of the care environment should be found if these rituals take place.

Dying and death

Roman Catholics may wish a priest to carry out the sacrament of the 'Last Rites or Extreme Unction' (anointing). If they are able, the individual may also wish to receive Holy Communion and confess their sins to the priest either before receiving Holy Communion or separately. There are no particular rituals associated with last offices (the preparation of the deceased for burial).

Jehovah's Witnesses

Jehovah's Witnesses consider their religion to be a restoration of original first-century Christianity. They accept both the Old and the New Testament of the Bible as inspired by God. They believe in one God 'Jehovah', with the commands in the Bible being very important, and they therefore try to live by them at all times.

Considerations for practice

Jehovah's Witnesses are totally opposed to taking blood or blood products into the body. This means that they will not accept blood transfusions even in life-threatening situations. However, they may accept alternative treatments.

Diet

Anything that contains blood or blood products is unacceptable, as is meat that has come from an animal that has been strangled, shot or not bled properly. If in doubt, Jehovah's Witnesses should be offered a vegetarian diet.

Patient confidentiality

Confidentiality must be maintained at all times and the patient's permission must be sought regarding what information they would like to be passed on to their family.

Death and dying

There are no particular rites and rituals associated with death and dying.

Hinduism

Originating in northern India, Hinduism is an amalgamation of many local faiths and is inextricably linked to culture and social structure. Hindus believe there is one God who can be worshipped and understood in many different forms. There is a belief in reincarnation in which the status and caste (hereditary or marital social class system) of each life is determined by the behaviour in the last life.

Hinduism does not have one leader, a unified code of conduct or creed. Because of this diversity it is difficult to generalise about what a specific individual might believe.

Considerations for practice

Physical examination

Generally, Hindu patients will have a strong preference for being treated and cared for by healthcare staff of the same gender. Privacy during any procedure is very important and female patients may be reluctant to remove clothing. They may also wish for a family member to act as a chaperone when physical examination and procedures are being carried out. Care must be taken not to remove any jewellery, threads, etc. without the permission of the patient/family, as they often have a religious significance.

Personal hygiene

Hindus prefer to shower rather than bathe and should always be provided with water for washing when they go to the toilet.

Diet

Most Hindus are vegetarian, refusing to take the lives of animals for food. Devout Hindus would not eat off a plate on which meat has been served so an acceptable alternative (for example a disposable plate) might need to be found.

Medication

Medication that contains animal products should be avoided.

Family and individual

As Hindus are intimately integrated with their extended family, there may be issues related to decision-making. Often decisions may be taken by a senior member of the family, or a female patient may wish her husband to consent to any treatment on her behalf.

Hindu patients tend to be visited frequently by their extended family, which can cause some difficulties with regard to preset visiting times and the policies concerning numbers of visitors which exist in most hospitals. The family may also wish to perform religious ceremonies with the patient. Privacy should be afforded to allow this to happen.

Prayer and ritual observance

Devout Hindus pray three times a day (at sunrise, noon and sunset). They should be assisted to wash before prayers if they are unable to do so independently.

Where possible a quiet area should be provided and they should not be disturbed during prayer. Patients may wish to have statues or pictures of Gods at their bedside and these items need to be treated with great care and respect.

Dying and death

Death in hospital can cause considerable religious distress to a Hindu patient and their family. Therefore, many patients may have a strong desire, and should be allowed, to die at home. If in hospital they will need to be surrounded by their family who may wish to read passages from holy texts, say prayers with and for them, and perform required ceremonies.

After death real distress may be caused if a non-Hindu touches the body without wearing disposable gloves. Unless otherwise advised by the family, close the eyes and straighten the legs. Do not cut the hair, nails or beard. Hands should be placed on the chest with the palms together and fingers under the chin. Religious objects or jewellery should not be removed. Wrap the body in a plain white sheet.

Judaism

Jews consider themselves a nation as much as a religious community. The religious aspects of Judaism are based on the relationship between God and man, and relationships between individual humans based on principles of fairness and equality. Religious observance is a means of publicly displaying a personal acceptance of a close connection between the individual and God. Orthodox Jews are very devout in their faith and adhere strictly to the ancient Torah (holy scriptures/laws). Reform or Liberal Jews believe in the Torah but interpret the laws and scriptures in relation to modern-day circumstances.

Considerations for practice

Personal hygiene

Orthodox Jews may wish to wash themselves before and after eating. Running water is required for this, so if the patient is unable to get out of bed, a bowl and jug of water should be offered.

Diet

Only kosher food is acceptable to many Jewish patients. Milk and meat are not eaten at the same meal. Meat must be killed according to kosher ritual and is acceptable only from animals which chew the cud and have cloven hooves, or poultry. Pig and rabbit are forbidden. Fish must have fins and scales and therefore shellfish are forbidden. If kosher meals are not available, a vegetarian diet should be offered.

Prayer

Jews usually say prayers three times a day and privacy and peace should be given to allow this to happen. The Sabbath is a holy day in which Jews are restricted in what they may do. It begins at sunset on Friday and ends at sunset on Saturday. It is important to establish the patient's principles with regard to the Sabbath as they may significantly impact on the care offered during this time (for example, a patient may not be willing to use a pen to sign their name on forms).

Death and dying

A Jew who is dying may wish to hear or recite special psalms (particularly Psalm 23).

After death the body should be touched by care staff as little as possible and disposable gloves should be worn at all times. Contact should be made with either the next of kin or the rabbi as soon as possible, as they will arrange for the preparation of the body. The face should be covered with a clean cloth or sheet, arms should not be crossed but left at the side of the body with palms facing inwards. Any catheters, drains and tubes should be left in place, as should any wound dressings. Open wounds should be covered. If the patient dies at night the light should be left on when there is no one in the room or bed space. Female bodies should be attended to by female care staff and if at all possible male bodies by male care staff.

Islam

Islam means 'submission and peace' and includes acceptance of those articles of faith, commands and ordinances revealed through the prophet Mohammed. Muslims follow the Islamic faith and believe that the whole universe is under the direction of Allah and nothing can happen unless he wills it. Most practising Muslims follow five main duties or pillars of Islam:
- Have faith in one God
- Pray at five set times every day
- Give a required amount to charity each year
- Fast during the holy month of Ramadan
- Make a pilgrimage (hajj) once in their lives to Mecca, if they can.

Considerations for practice

Physical examination/procedures

Physical examination and procedures should generally be carried out by a member of the healthcare team of the same gender as the patient. Privacy during any procedure is very important and female patients may be reluctant to remove clothing. They may also wish for a family member to act as a chaperone when physical examination/procedures are being carried out. Consideration should be given to ensure that the patient remains covered appropriately throughout the examination and any other procedure that may need to be performed as part of the care provided. Care must be taken not to remove any jewellery without the permission of the patient/family, as it often has a special or religious significance to the patient.

Personal hygiene

In general Muslims prefer to wash in running water so a shower is preferable to a bath where possible.

Diet

Meat must be slaughtered according to the halal ritual, in which the meat is drained of blood. Halal beef, lamb and chicken are eaten but pork and foods containing blood are forbidden. Fish and eggs are allowed but must not be cooked where pork and other non-halal meat is cooked (for example in a hospital or care home kitchen). If halal food is not available the family should be allowed to bring food in for the patient, or a strict vegetarian diet should be offered. During the month of Ramadan a Muslim must fast between sunrise and sunset. Although Muslims who are temporarily ill or who have a chronic condition may be permitted not to fast, it is important for healthcare staff to understand that the fasting may still compromise medical diets, tests, etc.

Medication

Islam prohibits the consumption of alcohol so Muslims may refuse medication that contains alcohol.

Prayer

Devout Muslims will pray up to five times a day. Privacy and peace should be given to allow them to do this. Before prayer a ritual wash in running water is undertaken, in which face, hands and arms are washed in a predetermined way. If the patient is confined to bed they may need help with their preparation for prayer and a jug of water and a bowl will ensure a source of running water is available. Clothes should also be changed if they have become soiled. There is a special format for prayer that uses special hand gestures instead of whole body movements that can be carried out when the patient is confined to bed.

Family and individual

Muslim patients tend to be visited frequently by their extended family, which can cause some difficulties with regard to preset visiting times and the policies concerning numbers of visitors which exist in most hospitals. Many of the visitors may also wish to be involved in the care of the patient, so they should be advised on how they may contribute. As Muslims do not generally encourage men and women to mix freely in public, Muslim patients should not be placed in mixed wards.

Death and dying

As the person approaches death they will expect to have their family and friends around them, which can sometimes mean a considerable number of people visiting at any one time. If this happens, caring for the patient in a side room may be preferable. If members of the family are not in attendance when death occurs, healthcare staff should wear disposable gloves so that they do not directly touch the body. The person's head should be turned towards Mecca (usually southeast in the UK), the arms and legs straightened, eyes and mouth closed and the body covered entirely with a clean white sheet. Female bodies should be attended to by female care staff and, if at all possible, male bodies by male care staff. The remaining preparation of the body will be carried out by a member of the family, who should be contacted immediately – Islamic religious law calls for burial to take place as soon as possible, usually within 24 hours of death.

Sikhism

'Sikh' translates roughly as 'student or disciple' and originated as a reformist movement of Hinduism; its founder, Guru Nanak, attempting to combine the best features of Hinduism and Islam. Sikhs believe in one God and must live a spiritual life and develop their own individual relationship with God by dedicating their lives to doing good. Thus, while on this earth they should be truthful, gentle, kind and generous, and work towards the common good. Historically they perceived all men as equal, and more recently perceptions of men and women being equal are also prominent.

Sikhs have five 'signs' which they should wear at all times, known as the 'five Ks'.

They are:
- Kesh – uncut beard and hair;
- Kangha – wooden comb;
- Kara – a steel bracelet worn on the right wrist;
- Kirpan – a sharp knife with a double-edged blade (often now in the UK worn in the form of a badge or brooch);
- Kaccha – long underpants/trousers.

Considerations for practice

Physical examination

Generally Sikh men and women would prefer to be examined by a member of the healthcare staff of the same gender as themselves, and would wish to remain as covered as possible through an examination or procedure. Removal of any of the five Ks must be strictly with the agreement/permission of the patient or their family. When removed they should be treated with great care.

Personal hygiene

Sikhs prefer to use running water for washing and thus prefer to shower rather than bathe. If a patient is unable to use a shower, a bowl and a jug of water is an acceptable alternative. Male Sikhs may also need help to remove their turban (which has to be done at least once a day). Both men and women may need help with the required regular washing, drying and combing of their hair.

Diet

Meat that has been prepared in a ritualistic way for another religion should not be given to a Sikh. Although there are no specific rules about not eating meat, many Sikhs are vegetarian and this includes not eating fish or eggs.

Prayer

Sikhs spend a lot of time in meditative contemplation of God. Before prayers the person will want to wash themselves and dress in clean clothes if necessary. A patient may need help to ensure this happens.

Family and the individual

Visiting the sick is a duty of the Sikh community, so the patient may receive many visitors. Families and friends will also expect to be involved in discussions about treatment and the provision of healthcare. A patient may refuse treatment or care if the family does not agree with it. Sikh patients should not be placed in mixed wards.

Death and dying

If a member of the family is not available, healthcare staff should wear disposable gloves to avoid direct contact with the patient after death. Do not undress, wash the body or remove any of the five Ks, as that is something the family would wish to carry out themselves. Drains and other tubes can be removed. The body should then be wrapped in a clean white cloth/sheet ready for the family to care for.

Buddhism

Buddhism is a way of life rather than an organised religion. Its focus is on personal spiritual development and the attainment of a deeper insight into the true nature of life, rather than a set of ritualistic practices. It teaches that all life is interconnected and the path to enlightenment is through the practice and development of morality, meditation and wisdom. The practice of Buddhism is extremely diverse and Buddhists from different regions will have different interpretations of the central ideas.

Considerations for practice

Diet

Most Buddhists tend to be vegetarians.

Medication

Some Buddhists may refuse to accept medication that contains alcohol or animal products. Some may prefer to use other strategies, such as meditation, to relieve pain as an alternative to conventional analgesia.

Dying

A Buddhist who knows that they are dying will probably wish to have their family and friends with them to meditate and chant mantras as death approaches. They will need as much peace and quiet as possible to allow this to happen. After death, do not touch or move the body of a Buddhist patient until advice has been sought from an appropriate source (for example, the family, friends or the hospital chaplain).

(Neusner, 2010; Weller, 2001; Henley and Schott, 1999; www.ethnicityonline.net)

CHAPTER SUMMARY

- Culture encompasses the values, beliefs, behaviour, practices and material objects that constitute a people's way of life.
- The Human Rights Act (1998) and the Equality Act (2010) are the two main pieces of legislation relating to cultural awareness that you need to be familiar with.
- Everyone in health and social care provision should make sure that they deliver culturally sensitive care that not only meets the religious, dietary and linguistic requirements of patients but also ensures that the principle of person-centred care is preserved.
- Cultural awareness requires self-awareness, knowledge and sensitivity.

Further information

Further reading and information on a range of religions and implications for practice in respect of healthcare can be obtained from the internet. Your starting point could include www.interfaith. org.uk and www.bbc.co.uk/religion/religions.

References

Andrews, M. and Boyle, J. (2015) *Transcultural Concepts in Nursing Care*, 7th edition. Philadelphia, PA: Wolters Kluwer.

Department for Constitutional Affairs (2006) *A Guide to the Human Rights Act 1998*, 3rd edition. London: DCA. Available from https://webarchive.nationalarchives.gov.uk/+/http:/www.dca.gov.uk/peoples-rights/human-rights/pdf/act-studyguide.pdf (accessed 2 May 2019)

Department of Health and NHS Commissioning Board (2012) *Compassion in Practice. Nursing, Midwifery and Care Staff, Our Vision and Strategy*. London: DH and NHS Commissioning Board.

Equality and Human Rights Commission (2017) *An Introduction to the Equality Act 2010*. Available at: www.equality-humanrights.com/en/equality-act-2010/what-equality-act (accessed 4 April 2019)

Giger, J. (2017) *Transcultural Nursing: assessment and intervention*, 7th edition. St Louis, MO: Elsevier.

Henley, A. and Schott, J. (1999) *Culture, Religion and Patient Care in a Multi-Ethnic Society: a handbook for professionals*. London: Age Concern Books.

Hofstede, G., Hofstede, G.J. and Minkov, M. (2010) *Cultures and Organizations: software of the mind*, 3rd edition. New York: McGraw-Hill.

Human Rights Act (1998) Available at: www.equalityhumanrights.com/en/human-rights/human-rights-act (accessed 4 April 2019)

Jirwe, M. (2008) *Cultural Competence in Nursing*. Stockholm: Karolinska Institute. Available at: https://openarchive.ki.se/xmlui/handle/10616/39797 (accessed 8 April 2019)

Klein, E. (1971) *A Comprehensive Etymological Dictionary of the English Language*. Amsterdam: Elsevier Scientific Publishing Co.

Macionis, J. and Plummer, K. (2011) *Sociology: a global introduction*, 5th edition. Harlow: Prentice Hall.

McFarland, M. and Wehbe-Alamah, H. (2018) *Leininger's Transcultural Nursing: concepts, theories, research & practice*, 4th edition. New York: McGraw-Hill.

Narayanasamy, A. (2002) The ACCESS model: a transcultural nursing practice framework. *British Journal of Nursing*, **11(9)**: 643–50.

Neusner, J. (ed.) (2010) *Introduction to World Religions: communities and culture*. Nashville, TN: Abingdon Press.

Northern Ireland Assembly (2013) Census 2011: *Detailed Characteristics of Ethnicity and Country of Birth at the Northern Ireland level*. Available at: www.niassembly.gov.uk/globalassets/documents/raise/publications/2013/general/13813.pdf (accessed 4 April 2019)

Nursing and Midwifery Council (2018a) *Future Nurse: standards of proficiency for registered nurses*. London: NMC.

Nursing and Midwifery Council (2018b) *The Code: professional standards of practice and behaviour for nurses, midwives and nursing associates*. London: NMC.

Office for National Statistics (2012) *Ethnicity and National Identity in England and Wales: 2011*. Available at: www.ons.gov.uk/peoplepopulationandcommunity/culturalidentity/ethnicity/articles/ethnicityandnationalidentityinenglandandwales/2012-12-11 (accessed 4 April 2019)

Papadopoulos, I. (ed.) (2006) *Transcultural Health and Social Care: development of culturally competent practitioners*. Edinburgh: Churchill Livingstone.

Scottish Government (2012) *Ethnic Group Demographics*. Available at: www.gov.scot/Topics/People/Equality/Equalities/DataGrid/Ethnicity/EthPopMig (accessed 4 April 2019)

Walsh, M. (2018) *Key Topics in Social Sciences: an A–Z guide for student nurses*. Banbury: Lantern Publishing Ltd.

Weller, P. (ed.) (2001) *Religions in the UK: a multi-faith directory*, 3rd edition. Derby: University of Derby.

Useful websites

www.bihr.org.uk/my-human-rights?gclid=CNi0pqiQ7csCFRS6GwodpgEHLQ (accessed 8 April 2019)
www.ethnicity-facts-figures.service.gov.uk/ (accessed 8 April 2019)
www.gov.uk (accessed 8 April 2019)
www.gov.uk/government/organisations/department-of-health/about/equality-and-diversity
(accessed 8 April 2019)

QUALITY CARE

The aim of this chapter is to introduce the quality care and quality assurance which guide healthcare provision in the UK and, in particular, in England.

LEARNING OUTCOMES

On completion of this chapter you should be able to:
- understand some of the main policies and procedures which inform and guide quality in the provision of healthcare
- briefly outline the concepts of clinical governance and clinical audit
- understand issues relevant to vulnerable adults
- understand the importance of patients' and service users' views in quality assurance
- briefly outline the key steps in the development of integrated care pathways

» Defining quality assurance

Quality assurance within the NHS is made up of three components: patient safety, patient experience and clinical effectiveness and these include:

Patient safety

- Care Quality Commission (CQC) registration of providers and quality monitoring visits
- Patient Safety Programmes
- Cleanliness and healthcare-associated infection (HCAI)
- Tissue viability
- Serious incident data
- Safeguarding children and adults and case analysis

- Patient safety thermometer
- Summary hospital mortality indicator (SHMI).

Patient experience

- National and local surveys
- PROMs (patient reported outcome measures)
- Friends and family scores
- Complaints and patient advice and liaison service (PALS) data
- Same-sex accommodation
- Procedure initiative
- Quality accounts
- Carer projects and involvement
- Quality impact assessments.

Clinical effectiveness

- National strategies
- National Institute for Health and Care Excellence (NICE) quality standards and guidelines
- NHS Quality and Outcomes Framework
- National and local clinical audits
- The Commissioning for Quality and Innovation (CQUIN) schemes
- Learning from national reports
- High impact innovations
- Quality schedules.

Therefore quality assurance is the maintenance of a desired level of quality in a service by means of attention to every stage of the process of delivery. Quality assurance is an ongoing, systematic comprehensive evaluation of healthcare services and the impact of those services; consequently it is defined as all activities undertaken to predict and prevent poor quality. Within the context of healthcare, Spath and Kelly (2017) explore how quality assurance aims to continuously improve quality and safety for those who come in contact with health services, and aims to ensure that those services are current and lead to desirable health outcomes. Joshi *et al.* (2014) suggest that for healthcare professionals, quality assurance is essentially about delivering safe, effective, efficient, timely, patient-centred and equitable care.

>> Care quality assurance is the maintenance of a desired level of care by means of attention to every stage of the process of care delivery.

>> A brief history of the organisation of quality assurance in UK healthcare

Before the 1980s	Quality assurance in the health service tended to be implicit rather than explicit. According to Dowding and Barr (2002), this was largely due to the fact that healthcare was felt to exist for altruistic motives rather than for profit, and these motives were not open to quality scrutiny.
	International influences led in **1984** to the British government launching the National Quality Campaign for both public and private industries, and within this the National Health Service (NHS) was strongly encouraged to ensure quality control systems were in place.
By the 1990s	Specific requirements and advice on quality were being set out in government health policy. For example, The Patients' Charter (Department of Health, 1991) set down precise national standards regarding various rights and expectations for all patients.
	Subsequent policy and legislation, including *A First Class Service: improving quality in the new NHS* (Department of Health, 1998), made more specific plans for progress in improving the health service, especially in terms of effectiveness, efficiency and excellence. These plans reflected the need for clear lines of responsibility and quality management activities incorporating monitoring and continuous improvement. *A First Class Service* also identified clinical effectiveness, evidence-based practice, clinical supervision and continuing professional development activities as specific requirements for healthcare practitioners in support of quality assurance.
Since 2000	There have been a number of initiatives and policies, including the *Equity and Excellence: liberating the NHS* White Paper (Department of Health, 2010a), which have identified successive governments' commitment to continually trying to improve quality of care; and NHS Improvement (2016) who support providers to minimise patient safety incidents and drive improvements in safety and quality.

>> National quality assurance

In the UK, health service quality processes can take place at both national and local level. There is no easy way to introduce you to the plethora of organisations, agencies and initiatives with a mandate to ensure quality of care provision at each of these levels. However, you need to have a basic understanding/awareness of the key agencies, as you will encounter their work either directly or indirectly in nursing practice.

Care Quality Commission (CQC)

The CQC began operating on 1 April 2009 as the independent regulator of all health and adult social care services in England, including those provided by the NHS, local authorities, private companies and voluntary organisations. By law all health and adult social care providers (including the NHS) must be registered with the CQC. This also includes primary medical services and general practitioners. Without registration, providers are not allowed to operate. The Commission is funded through a combination of registration fee income and government grant-in-aid.

>> The role of the CQC is to ensure that the care provided to people meets the government standards of quality and safety.

The role of the CQC is to ensure that the care provided in hospitals, dental surgeries and those of general practitioners (GPs), ambulances, care homes and other services to people in their own homes and elsewhere meets the government standards of quality and safety. It also protects the interests of people detained under the Mental Health Act.

The Commission carries out its role mainly by the process of inspection. Regular checks are carried out on health and social care services. These are known as *comprehensive inspections* and are used to make sure services are providing care that is safe, caring, effective, responsive to people's needs and well led. Comprehensive inspections are usually announced in advance.

The CQC also carries out *focused inspections* which may not be announced in advance. These are smaller in scale than comprehensive inspections, although they follow a similar process. Focused inspections are carried out for two reasons:
- to look at something the Commission is concerned about, which might have been raised during a comprehensive inspection or through their monitoring work
- if there is a change in a care provider's circumstances; for example, in the organisation – they may have been involved in a takeover, a merger or an acquisition.

An important part of the Commission's work is collecting data from service users' experiences of care services. In some cases it involves patients and their carers directly in working alongside its inspectors to give an expert user view of services.

It also makes use of all informal and formal information and data to monitor what is happening inside health and social care systems, as well as across both health and social care, in order to identify where a pattern of incidents indicates that something untoward may be happening.

If a provider is not meeting the government standards of quality and safety then the Commission has a range of legal powers and duties to enforce the appropriate standards. These include:
- issuing a warning notice requiring improvements within a set period of time
- issuing fixed penalty notices, suspending or cancelling the service's registration
- prosecution.

In order to enforce the standards, the Commission is able, depending on the circumstances, to liaise with other agencies including local authorities, regulatory bodies such as Monitor and Healthwatch (see below), NHS England and other inspectorates including Ofsted and HMI Prisons. They also liaise with professional regulators such as the NMC.

The CQC does not have a remit in Scotland, Northern Ireland or Wales. These each have their own similar regulatory bodies. In Scotland this is the Care Inspectorate; in Northern Ireland, the Regulation and Quality Improvement Authority; and in Wales, Healthcare Inspectorate Wales.

NHS Improvement (NHSI)

NHSI is responsible for overseeing Foundation Trusts and NHS Trusts, as well as independent providers that provide NHS-funded care. It supports providers to give patients consistently safe, high quality, compassionate care within local health systems that are financially sustainable. It was established in April 2016 and merged several organisations such as Monitor, NHS Trust Development Authority, Patient Safety (from NHS England), National Reporting and Learning System, Advancing Change Team and Intensive Support Teams all focused on quality improvement.

Monitor

Monitor has a duty to set prices, enable integrated care, safeguard patient choice and prevent anti-competitive behaviour and support commissioners to protect essential healthcare services, and has been part of NHS Improvement since 2016.

ACTIVITY 6.1

Access NHS Improvement (using the link below or QR code on the right) and explore who they are and what they do. Choose one of the 'themes' such as Patient Safety, access one of the improvement tools and make your own notes on how this is used in practice.

https://improvement.nhs.uk/improvement-hub/

The Health and Safety Executive (HSE)

The Health and Safety Executive (HSE) is the national independent watchdog for work-related health, safety and illness. It acts in the public interest to reduce work-related death and serious injury across Great Britain's workplaces. This includes private or publicly owned health and social care settings throughout the UK.

The HSE does not normally investigate issues of clinical judgement or matters that relate to the quality of care provided. However, it does take the lead on employee health and safety and may also deal with non-clinical risks to patients (for example trips, falls, scalding, electrical safety, etc.). It also deals with aspects of risk that apply to both staff and patients (for example manual handling). In order to fulfil its role the HSE works in partnership with co-regulators in local authorities to inspect, investigate and where necessary take enforcement action. As at 2018, HSE inspectors have the power to:

- enter premises
- inspect and investigate
- take measurements, samples and photographs
- require an area or machine to be left undisturbed
- seize, render harmless or destroy dangerous items
- obtain information and take statements.

(www.hse.gov.uk)

NHS complaints procedure

Every NHS organisation has a complaints procedure. If a patient, or someone acting on behalf of the patient or person with their consent, wants to complain about an NHS service they can ask for a copy, which explains what needs to be done. Complaints may be made in writing, by email or verbally. The NHS complaints procedure covers complaints made by a patient or person about any matter connected with the provision of NHS services by NHS organisations or primary care practitioners (GPs, dentists, opticians and pharmacists).

The procedure also covers services provided overseas and by the private sector, where the NHS has paid for them.

If an individual is dissatisfied with the treatment or service they have received from the NHS they are entitled to make a complaint, have it considered, and receive a response from the NHS organisation or primary care practitioner concerned. The complaint must normally be made within 12 months of the event or within 12 months of becoming aware that the person has something to complain about. These time limits can be waived if there is good reason to do so.

Under the NHS Constitution an individual making a complaint has the right to:
- have their complaint dealt with efficiently, and properly investigated
- know the outcome of any investigation into their complaint
- take the complaint to the Independent Parliamentary and Health Service Ombudsman if they are not satisfied with the way the NHS has dealt with the complaint
- make a claim for a judicial review if they think they have been directly affected by an unlawful act or decision of an NHS body
- receive compensation if they have been harmed.

(Department of Health, 2015b)

The first stage of the procedure is known as 'local resolution', with the complaint, in the first instance, being made to the organisation or primary care practitioner who provided the services. Initially this may be by voicing concerns to a member of staff or the Patient Advice and Liaison Service (PALS). However, if the individual wishes to make the complaint more formal, they can do so either orally or in writing (including by email) to the organisation's complaints manager.

If the individual is not satisfied with the response to their complaint they can request or agree to an 'independent review' of their case through the Health Service Ombudsman. This is an independent body set up to investigate complaints about health services and promote improvements of healthcare as a result. Financial compensation, legal action and professional misconduct are not dealt with through this process.

RECAP

- Various organisations are responsible for ensuring the quality of care, including the CQC, NHS Improvement, Monitor and the HSE.
- Everyone has the right to complain if they are not happy with the service they have received from the NHS and to have the complaint dealt with efficiently and investigated properly.

FURTHER READING
Further information on monitoring and promoting improvement of quality of healthcare in Wales, Scotland and Northern Ireland can be obtained from:
Wales: www.hiw.org.uk
Scotland: www.healthcareimprovementscotland.org
Northern Ireland: www.dhsspsni.gov.uk

›› Local clinical level

Quality assurance at local level covers a variety of activities including clinical audit, patients' and users' views and patient advisory services. Further issues such as safeguarding, integrated care pathways (ICPs) (Middleton *et al.*, 2001) and the *Essence of Care* (Department of Health, 2010b) initiative can also be included here. An ICP is a person-centred and evidence-based framework which tells multidisciplinary and multi-agency care providers, service users and their carers what should be expected at any point along the care journey. *Essence of Care* supports localised quality improvement, by providing a set of established and refreshed benchmarks supporting front-line care across care settings at a local level.

Clinical governance

Clinical governance describes the structures, processes and culture needed to ensure that healthcare organisations – and all individuals within them – can assure the quality of the care they provide and are continuously seeking to improve it. Since the term was first introduced (in 1998), it has been recognised that these structures and processes should be fully integrated with other aspects of the governance of healthcare organisations, including their financial, information and research governance (Public Health England, 2015).

Covering the organisation's systems and processes for monitoring and improving services, the key elements of clinical governance include:
- strong leadership and accountability
- patient, public, carer consultation and involvement
- clinical effectiveness and commitment to quality
- clinical audit
- education, training and continuous professional development
- research and development
- clinical risk management
- staff management and performance
- health staff having accountability for clinical quality
- use of information about patients' experiences, outcomes and processes.

All of the key elements are of equal value and importance and all are interrelated.

In principle, clinical governance is perceived as being about ensuring safe, high quality care from those involved in a patient's journey, while ensuring the patient remains the main focus and priority.

Clinical audit

Clinical audit is an essential and integral part of clinical governance at local level. Clinical audit is a way to find out if healthcare is being provided in line with standards and it lets care providers and patients know where their service is doing well, and where there could be improvements.

The National Institute for Health and Care Excellence (NICE) describes it as:

> *"... a process for monitoring standards of clinical care to see if it is being carried out in the best way possible (known as 'best practice'). Clinical audit can be described as a systematic 'cycle'. It involves measuring care against specific criteria, taking action to improve it if necessary, and monitoring the process to sustain improvement. As the process continues, an even higher level of quality is achieved."*

(NICE, 2012)

Essentially, clinical audit is about clinical effectiveness and quality improvement and is now a key component of the clinical governance framework and well established both within the NHS and the independent sector.

The key elements of clinical audit are:
- setting standards/criteria for a chosen area/topic
- measuring current practice
- comparing the results with the standards/criteria set
- changing practice if required
- re-auditing to ensure quality practice has been maintained or practice has improved.

Put together, these elements are usually referred to as the 'audit cycle', as shown in *Figure 6.1.*

The fundamental principles associated with clinical audit are that it should:
- be professionally led
- be viewed as an educational process
- be a routine part of clinical practice
- be based on the setting of standards
- generate results based on the setting of standards
- generate results that can be used to improve outcome of quality care

- involve management in both the process and outcome of audit
- be confidential at the individual patient/clinician level
- be informed by the views of patients/clients.

(NICE, 2012; Burgess, 2011)

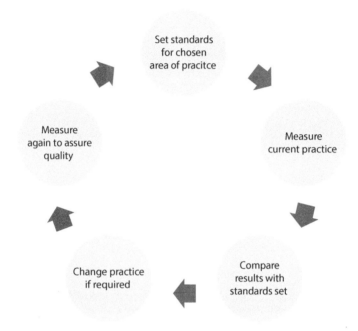

Figure 6.1: *The audit cycle.*

The views of patients and service users

Since the early 2000s there has been a clear policy move towards a culture of regularly involving and consulting patients and the public in decision-making and service improvement. In 2003 the Health and Social Care Act placed a duty on the NHS to engage actively with community and service users. In October 2008 this was taken a stage further when the government published the Local Government and Public Health Act (Department of Health, 2008). This Act contained new duties for health organisations to reinforce and improve the way the NHS pays attention to and utilises the views of the public to improve local health services.

Healthwatch

The Health and Social Care Act (Department of Health, 2012) provided for the establishment of Healthwatch England as an independent consumer champion for both health and social care. Healthwatch England is part of a Healthwatch network which seeks to give a more powerful voice, both locally and nationally, to the key issues that affect people who use health and social care services.

Views from all sections of the community are sought and it functions at two levels:

Healthwatch England

Healthwatch England works at a national level:
- providing leadership, support and advice to local Healthwatch organisations
- gathering and analysing information provided by local Healthwatch organisations
- ensuring the views of people who use health and social care services are relayed to the Secretary of State, the CQC, the NHS Commissioning Board, Monitor and all local authorities in England.

Local Healthwatch organisations

The role of local Healthwatch organisations includes:
- being able to influence how services are set up and commissioned, by having a seat on the local health and wellbeing board
- providing information, advice and support about local services
- providing information and recommendations to Healthwatch England and the CQC
- being based in and funded by Local Authorities.

(Local Government Association, 2013)

In Scotland the equivalent is the Scottish Health Council; in Wales it is Community Health Councils and in Northern Ireland it is the Patient and Client Council.

The Patient Advice and Liaison Service (PALS)

Established throughout the NHS, this service offers confidential support and advice directly to service users, families and carers if they have a perceived cause for complaint or concern. Although not part of the complaints procedure itself, the service liaises with staff, managers and, where appropriate, other relevant organisations, to negotiate informally and encourage fast solution of the problem or concern. The core functions of PALS are to:
- be identifiable and accessible to patients, their carers, friends and families
- provide on-the-spot help in every Trust, with the power to negotiate immediate solutions or speedy resolution of problems
- act as a gateway to appropriate independent advice and advocacy support from local and national sources

- provide accurate information to patients, carers and families, about the Trust's services, and about other health-related issues
- act as a catalyst for change and improvement by providing the Trust with information and feedback on problems arising and gaps in services
- operate within a local network with other PALS in their area and work across organisational boundaries
- support staff at all levels within the Trust to develop a responsive culture.

(NHS, 2018)

RECAP

- Clinical governance describes the structures, processes and culture needed to assure the quality of the care provided. Clinical audit is an essential part of clinical governance at local level.
- Patients' and users' views are an important factor in assuring quality care. Local Healthwatch organisations influence care services by having a seat on the local health and wellbeing board. PALS offers confidential advice and support to care service users.

» Further aspects of quality assurance

Safeguarding children and young people and vulnerable adults

Everyone has a right to feel safe, and to live without fear of abuse, neglect or exploitation. Safeguarding was explored in *Chapter 3*, and one purpose of the quality care and assurance process outlined above is to ensure action is taken to promote the welfare of children and protect them from harm. Safeguarding also exists to ensure that vulnerable adults are not abused

> » Safeguarding is everyone's responsibility.

by being mistreated, neglected or harmed by another person who holds a position of trust. Safeguarding is everyone's responsibility and involves consistently providing safe and effective care and taking action where necessary to ensure the best outcomes (Berwick, 2013).

Following a number of high profile serious incidents involving vulnerable adults, the Department of Health published *No Secrets: guidance on developing and implementing multi-agency policies and procedures to protect vulnerable adults from abuse* (Department of Health, 2015a). This document provides guidance on actions to be taken within health and social care regarding the appropriate protection and support of vulnerable adults. The aim of the guidance has been to construct a framework in which all relevant agencies are required to work together to ensure strong and coherent policies and procedures are in place, and implemented locally for the protection of vulnerable adults who are at risk of abuse. Abuse in this context is defined by the Department of Health (Department of Health, 2015a, p. 9) as "a violation of an individual's human and civil rights by another person or persons".

The abuse may be a single or repeated act, may occur in any relationship and may result in serious harm to, or exploitation of, the person subjected to it. The main forms of abuse can be identified as:

- **physical abuse** (includes misuse of medication and restraint)
- **sexual abuse**
- **psychological abuse** (includes verbal abuse, controlling and withdrawal from services or supportive networks, coercion)
- **financial/material abuse** (includes theft, fraud and misuse or misappropriation of possessions)
- **neglect and acts of omission** (includes ignoring medical or physical care needs and withholding necessities of life such as medication and adequate nutrition)
- **discriminatory abuse** (includes racist, sexist and ageist abuse and harassment).

A further form of abuse, referring specifically to neglect and poor professional practice, is often referred to as 'institutional abuse'. This ranges from an isolated event of poor or unsatisfactory professional practice through to ongoing ill treatment or gross misconduct.

The NMC defines abuse in the registrant–client relationship as "the result of the misuse of power or a betrayal of trust, respect or intimacy between the registrant and the client, which the registrant should know would cause physical or emotional harm to the client" (NMC, 2002, p. 7). Its guidance identifies zero tolerance of abuse as the only philosophy consistent with protecting the public. It stresses that registrants have a responsibility to ensure that they safeguard the interests of their clients at all times and to protect patients/service users from all forms of abuse.

>> All nurses, including students, must safeguard the interests of their patients and protect them from all forms of abuse.

If, in the course of their professional practice, registrants suspect or believe that a client is being, or has been abused, they must report this as soon as practical to a person of appropriate authority. This zero tolerance of abuse is also expected from students of nursing.

In 2015 the NMC published the guidelines *Raising Concerns* (NMC, 2015). The guidance is for all nurses, midwives and nursing associates, and pre-registration nursing and midwifery students, no matter where they work. The document makes it clear that a nurse, midwife or nursing associate has a professional duty to put the interests of the people in their care first and to act to protect them if they consider they may be at risk. The purpose of the guidance is to establish principles for best practice in the raising of any concerns, which includes whistleblowing. It also explains the process that should be followed when raising concerns (pages 6–7 for students), whilst providing information about legislation in this area and indicating where confidential support and advice may be accessed.

It is advised that the guidance supports, and should be read together with, *The Code: professional standards of practice and behaviour for nurses, midwives and nursing associates* (NMC, 2018), and in conjunction with local-based policies with regard to the protection of vulnerable adults.

ACTIVITY 6.2

Access, read and keep a copy of the guidelines *Raising Concerns: guidance for nurses, midwives and nursing associates* from www.nmc.org.uk or by using the QR code on the right. Find out who the appropriate person is to raise concerns with in your institution and in your practice placement, and make a note of any specific procedure that applies.

Essence of Care

The *Essence of Care* benchmarks are a tool to help healthcare practitioners take a patient-focused and structured approach to sharing and comparing practice. They were also designed to support measures to improve quality, and to contribute to clinical governance within organisations. *Essence of Care 2010* (Department of Health, 2010b) supports and reflects a number of the themes in *Equity and Excellence: liberating the NHS* (Department of Health, 2010a). It focuses on what might be described as the fundamental and essential aspects of care, and it seeks to enable healthcare personnel to work with patients to identify best practice and to develop action plans to improve the quality of care and the experience of people who use care services.

It can be used by individuals, teams, directorates, and within and across organisations of all sizes. It can also be used locally or strategically, or ideally, both.

Benchmarking tools

In the context of *Essence of Care 2010* (Department of Health, 2010b) a benchmark is "a standard of best practice and care by which current practice and care is assessed or measured" (Department of Health, 2010b, p. 9).

Following from this, benchmarking is "a systematic process in which current practice and care are compared to, and amended to attain, best practice and care" (Department of Health, 2010b, p. 9).

The *Essence of Care 2010* (Department of Health, 2010b) benchmarks comprise:
- an overall person-focused outcome that expresses what people and carers want from care in a particular area of practice
- definitions of terms as appropriate
- general indicators, or goals, for best practice
- a number of factors, or topics, that need to be considered in order to achieve the overall person-focused outcome.

Each factor consists of:
- a person-focused statement of best practice and care which is placed at the extreme right of the continuum
- a statement of poor practice and care which is placed at the extreme left of the continuum
- indicators, or goals, identified by people, carers, association representatives and staff that support the attainment of best practice and care.

Patients, carers and professionals worked together to agree and describe person-focused outcomes, specific factors and indicators within the benchmarks in twelve areas of care:
- personal hygiene
- respect and dignity
- food and nutrition
- self-care
- safety
- record-keeping
- prevention and management of pain
- prevention and management of pressure ulcers
- bladder, bowel and continence care
- communication (between patients, carers and healthcare personnel)
- promoting health and wellbeing
- care environment.

All the sets of benchmarks are interrelated (Department of Health, 2010b).

Using clinical benchmarks

Essence of Care 2010 benchmarking is a systematic process intended to help health and social care organisations, teams or individual staff to achieve best practice and care. Changes and improvements focus on the indicators, or goals, within the factors, since these are the items that people, carers and staff believe are important for achieving best practice and care.

Briefly, the steps involved are:

STEP ONE	• establish priorities for improving practice and care within the environment or organisation
STEP TWO	• establish and agree best (evidence-based) practice and care for people within the organisation
STEP THREE	• ascertain current practice and care
STEP FOUR	• compare the differences, and identify the gaps and barriers, between current and best practice and care, and identify achievements
STEP FIVE	• develop a plan of what goals need to be met to achieve best practice and care, i.e. work out what needs to be done and how
STEP SIX	• implement the plan (i.e. change things; for example, activity, perspective, approach, culture, education and training, environment) to meet the goals
STEP SEVEN	• evaluate practice and care by assessing and measuring whether goals have been met
STEP EIGHT	• establish improved practice and care across a team or organisation(s)
STEP NINE	• establish priorities and further goals to continuously improve quality of practice and care, i.e. go through the steps again

The benchmarks are relevant to all health and social care settings. Therefore, the *Essence of Care* is presented in a generic format in order that it can be used in, for example, primary, secondary and tertiary settings and with all patient and/or carer groups, such as in paediatric care, mental health, cancer care, surgery and medicine (Department of Health, 2010b).

RECAP

- Safeguarding is a vital aspect of providing quality care, and the NMC's guidance identifies zero tolerance of abuse as the only philosophy consistent with protecting the public.
- *Essence of Care* benchmarks are a tool to help healthcare practitioners take a patient-focused and structured approach to sharing and comparing practice and to support measures to improve quality.

ACTIVITY 6.3

It is very important that you understand *Essence of Care* as you will no doubt be involved at some point in its implementation, whilst working both as a student nurse and as a qualified practitioner. Access and read the full document at www.dh.gov.uk or by using the QR code on the right. When you are next on practice placement, make a note of any areas you think might be priorities for improving practice.

CHAPTER SUMMARY

- Quality assurance is essentially about delivering safe, effective, efficient, timely, patient-centred and equitable care.
- In the UK, health service quality processes can take place at both national and local level.
- At local level, quality assurance covers a variety of activities including clinical governance, clinical audit, patients' and service users' views and patient advisory services.
- The protection of vulnerable adults, integrated care pathways and the *Essence of Care* initiatives can also be included in the processes.

Further information

Department for Education (2003) *Every Child Matters*. London: HMSO.

Department of Health (2012) *Protection of Freedom Act*. London: DH.

Department of Health (2014) *Introducing the Statutory Duty of Candour: a consultation on proposals to introduce a new CQC registration regulation*. London: DH.

Francis, R. (2013) *Report of the Mid Staffordshire NHS Foundation Trust Public Inquiry*. London: The Stationery Office.

Keogh, B. (2013) *Review into the Quality of Care and Treatment Provided by 14 Hospital Trusts in England*. London: NHS.

References

Berwick, D. (2013) *A Promise to Learn – A Commitment to Act: improving the safety of patients in England*. London: DH.

Burgess, R. (ed.) (2011) *New Principles of Best Practice in Clinical Audit*, 2nd edition. London: Radcliffe Publishing.

Department of Health (1991) *The Patient's Charter*. London: HMSO.

Department of Health (1998) *A First Class Service: improving quality in the new NHS*. London: DH.

Department of Health (2008) Local Government and Public Health Act. London: DH.

Department of Health (2010a) *Equity and Excellence: liberating the NHS*. London: DH.

Department of Health (2010b) *Essence of Care*. London: DH.

Department of Health (2012) The Health and Social Care Act 2012. London: DH.

Department of Health (2015a) *No Secrets: guidance on developing and implementing multi-agency policies and procedures to protect vulnerable adults from abuse.* London: DH.

Department of Health (2015b) *The NHS Constitution: the NHS belongs to us.* London: DH.

Dowding, L. and Barr, J. (2002) *Managing in Healthcare: a guide for nurses, midwives and health visitors.* Harlow: Pearson Education.

Joshi, M., Ransom, E., Nash, D. and Ransom, S. (eds) (2014) *The Healthcare Quality Book: vision, strategy and tools*, 3ʳᵈ edition. Chicago: Health Administration Press.

Local Government Association (2013) Available at: www.healthwatch.co.uk (accessed 8 May 2019)

Middleton, S., Barnett, J. and Reeves, D. (2001) *What is an Integrated Care Pathway?* Hayward Medical Communications. Available at: www.bandolier.org.uk/booth/glossary/ICP.html (accessed 7 April 2019)

National Institute for Clinical Excellence (NICE) (2012) *Methods for the Development of NICE Public Health Guidance*, 3rd edition. Available at: www.nice.org.uk/process/pmg4/chapter/introduction (accessed 3 June 2019)

NHS (2018) *Patient Advice and Liaison Service.* Available at: www.nhs.uk/common-health-questions/nhs-services-and-treatments/what-is-pals-patient-advice-and-liaison-service/ (accessed 7 April 2019)

NHS Improvement (England) (2016) *Freedom to Speak up: raising concerns (whistleblowing) policy for the NHS*. Available at: https://improvement.nhs.uk/uploads/documents/whistleblowing_ policy_30march.pdf (accessed 7 April 2019)

Nursing and Midwifery Council (2002) *Practitioner–client Relationships and the Prevention of Abuse.* London: NMC. Available at: www.brief-encounters.org/download/practitioner-client-relationships-and-the-prevention-of-abuse-nmc/ (accessed 13 May 2019)

Nursing and Midwifery Council (2015) *Raising Concerns: guidance for nurses, midwives and nursing associates.* Available at: www.nmc.org.uk/standards/guidance/raising-concerns-guidance-for-nurses-and-midwives (accessed 7 April 2019)

Nursing and Midwifery Council (2018) *The Code: professional standards of practice and behaviour for nurses, midwives and nursing associates.* Available at: www.nmc.org.uk/globalassets/sitedocuments/nmc-publications/nmc-code.pdf (accessed 9 April 2019)

Public Health England (2015) *Guidance: 4. Clinical governance.* Available at: https://www.gov.uk/government/publications/newborn-hearing-screening-programme-nhsp-operational-guidance/4-clinical-governance (accessed 2 May 2019)

Spath, P. and Kelly, D. (2017) *Applying Quality Management in Healthcare: a systems approach*, 4ᵗʰ edition. Chicago: Health Administration Press.

EVIDENCE-BASED PRACTICE

The aim of this chapter is to remind you about the importance of under-standing research and evidence-based practice as it underpins your nursing role every day in ensuring that you provide safe and effective care, both as a nursing student and when you are a registered nurse with the NMC.

LEARNING OUTCOMES

On completion of this chapter you should be able to:
- understand the concept of evidence-based practice
- appreciate the need to consider the evidence base when carrying out nursing care and issues related to its implementation

» Introduction

Historically nursing and, specifically, clinical procedures were based on rituals and traditions rather than research (Dougherty and Lister, 2015). An example of this was the use of egg white and oxygen in the 1970s to treat small pressure ulcers. However, since the 1990s, the term 'evidence-based practice' has become commonplace within the nursing profession, as nurses are required to justify the decisions they make and the care they deliver.

Evidence-based practice in nursing has evolved from the concept of evidence-based medicine. Sackett *et al.* (2000, p. 2) defined this as "the conscientious and explicit use of current best evidence in making decisions about the healthcare of patients". Subsequently, many authors have sought to define the specific meaning of evidence-based practice within nursing. For example:
- Cullum *et al.* (2008, p. 2) suggest that evidence-based nursing is "the application of valid, relevant, research-based information in nurse decision-making".
- Ingersoll (2000, p. 152) proposes that "evidence-based nursing practice is the conscientious, explicit and judicious use of theory-derived, research-based information in making decisions about care delivery to individuals or groups of patients with consideration of individual needs and preferences".

- Aveyard and Sharp's (2013, p. 4) definition also identifies the importance of the patient/service user's perspective: "[Evidence-based nursing] is practice that is supported by a clear, up-to-date rationale, taking into account the patient/client's preferences and using your own judgement". This aligns with the concept of person-centred care and also relates directly to a nurse's responsibility and accountability, as set out in by the NMC *Code* (2018a).

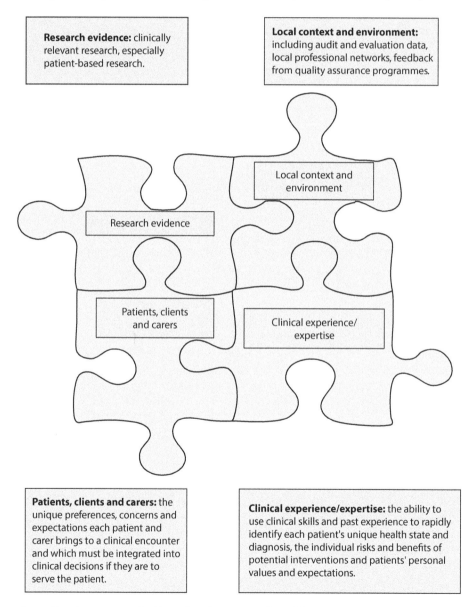

Research evidence: clinically relevant research, especially patient-based research.

Local context and environment: including audit and evaluation data, local professional networks, feedback from quality assurance programmes.

Local context and environment

Research evidence

Patients, clients and carers

Clinical experience/ expertise

Patients, clients and carers: the unique preferences, concerns and expectations each patient and carer brings to a clinical encounter and which must be integrated into clinical decisions if they are to serve the patient.

Clinical experience/expertise: the ability to use clinical skills and past experience to rapidly identify each patient's unique health state and diagnosis, the individual risks and benefits of potential interventions and patients' personal values and expectations.

Figure 7.1: *Components of evidence-based practice (adapted from Rycroft-Malone et al., 2004).*

Parahoo (2014) identifies a clear process for undertaking evidence-based practice. This includes identifying a question that relates to practice or policy, followed by searching for pertinent research studies which are analysed (appraised). After completing this, the findings from the identified studies are disseminated and implemented. Important skills for nurses to develop are not only the ability to undertake a systematic literature review but also to make "... use of evidence, clinical expertise and patients' views to make clinical decisions" (Parahoo, 2014, p. 393).

Figure 7.1 provides an example of the four key components of evidence-based practice and the relationship between them (from Rycroft-Malone *et al.*, 2004). This is covered in more detail later in this chapter.

In summary, the central principle of evidence-based practice is that nursing students, nurses and other health and social care practitioners combine their clinical or practice expertise and their knowledge of the client or patient with the high quality evidence from research (Sackett *et al.*, 1996). Heaslip and Lindsay (2018) emphasise that to provide the best possible care in practice, students must

>> Evidence-based practice bridges the gap between research and practice.

not only perform skilfully but also support their actions by referring to, and using, evidence; that is to say, practice is based on trustworthy data and factual information. Thus, evidence-based practice bridges the gap between research and practice.

>> Evidence-based practice in nursing

Nurses need to understand how information derived from research is turned into 'evidence' and thus informs practice. The NMC (2018a) clearly identifies that nurses have a responsibility to deliver care on the basis of the best evidence available and best practice. Thus, a nurse must:

- "make sure that any information or advice given is evidence-based including information relating to using any health care products or services", and
- "maintain the knowledge and skills you need for safe and effective practice".

Indeed, according to the *NHS Constitution for England* patients expect nurses not only to work in partnership with them but also that decisions about funding drugs and treatments "be made rationally following a proper consideration of the evidence" (NHS England, 2015, p. 7). See also: *Healthcare Principles* for Scotland; for Wales, *The Core Principles of NHS Wales* and for Northern Ireland, *The Charter for Patients and Clients*.

As already noted, evidence-based practice in nursing has its roots in the evidence-based medicine movement but in nursing, as we have seen, definitions of the term give prominence to the patients' views of effectiveness. The RCN (1996a) emphasised this by saying:

> "Evidence-based health care is rooted in the best scientific evidence and takes into account patients' views of effectiveness and clinical expertise in order to promote clinically effective services. This is essential in ensuring that health care practitioners do the things that work and are acceptable to patients, and do not do the things which don't work."
>
> (RCN, 1996a, cited in McClarey and Duff, 1997, p. 33)

Williamson *et al.* (2008) who developed the work of Bury and Mead (1998), identified the 'Six Rs of clinical effectiveness', as set out in *Figure 7.2*.

The right person	Was the person delivering the care competent, with the right skills and knowledge?
The right thing	Was there evidence to support the intervention, and was the patient agreeable?
The right way	Was an intervention used correctly, with correct skills and competence, or did it meet national guidelines and priorities?
The right place	Could the patient have been treated at home, or was there a more appropriate place based on specialist equipment or staff?
The right time	Was the intervention timely – would it have been more effective without a six-month wait?
The right result	Did it do what was intended?

Figure 7.2: *Six Rs of clinical effectiveness (Williamson* et al., *2008, adapted from Bury and Mead, 1998).*

More recently, the values and behaviours known as the 6Cs – Care, Compassion, Competence, Communication, Courage and Commitment (Cummings and Bennett, for the Department of Health, 2012) – underline the importance of implementing and delivering evidence-based practice. Within the 6Cs, it is recognised that patients/service users expect the right care to be given, that those caring are able to do the right thing and are competent to deliver care and treatments effectively based on evidence and research, and that there is a commitment to improve the care (see also *Chapter 3*).

Such statements by the RCN and the expected values and behaviours identified in the 6Cs highlight the importance of evidence-based practice in nursing. Parahoo (2014) points out that nurses represent the largest group of healthcare professionals throughout the world and spend considerably

>> Nurses spend considerably more time with patients than any other health professional group.

more time with patients than any other health professional group. Therefore, as a profession, nursing must build its body of knowledge and skills on solid evidence. However, Craig and Smyth (2012) issue a note of caution to this – the huge range of settings and people that nurses work with can be detrimental to implementing evidence-based practice; the settings in which nurses work are so varied that research cannot possibly be relevant to all. So, what is the right thing, and what are the choices available? Consequently, Craig and Smyth (2012) believe that the concept of evidence-based practice is particularly challenging for nurses.

Heaslip and Lindsay (2018, p. 4) outline what they consider the most important reasons for practice to be based on evidence:

- The public no longer trusts health and social care professionals to do what is best (consider the Francis Report of 2013 and the report on Gosport War Memorial Hospital of 2018).
- Professionals are conscious of the risk of being sued and want clear evidence for their practices.
- Emerging health and social care professions want to create their own evidence for their roles.
- Governments demand clear evidence before funding expensive new treatments or care strategies.

Evidence-based practice underlies all seven platforms of the NMC (2018b) *Future Nurse: standards of proficiency for registered nurses*. These standards set out the importance of applying research findings to "promote and inform best nursing practice" (ibid., Clause 1.7). This also means that evidence-based practice underpins all daily person-centred care/family-centred care. This is to ensure the delivery of clinically effective and safe treatments that improve the patient/service user's health outcomes in whatever field or areas of nursing you deliver care in. According to the NMC (2018b) a registered nurse is required to have "the confidence and ability to think critically, apply knowledge and skills, and provide expert, evidence-based, direct nursing care" (NMC, 2018b, p. 3). For nurses to deliver evidence-based practice, the NMC (2018b) clearly states that nurses need to be able to understand research methods as well as the ethics and governance processes involved in undertaking research. This is so they can "critically analyse, safely use, share and apply research findings to promote and inform best nursing practice" (ibid., Clause 1.7).

In addition the NMC (2018b, p. 16) states that registered nurses lead the provision of "evidence-based, compassionate and safe nursing" care and need to "ensure that [the] care they provide and delegate is person-centred and of a consistently high standard". As a nurse you will work in a range of care settings where you will need to "work in partnership with people, families and carers to evaluate whether care is effective and the goals of care have been met in line with their wishes, preferences and desired outcomes" (ibid., p. 16). This means that as a nurse you are required to:

- question
- critically appraise evidence
- take into account ethical considerations
- take into account the individual preferences of the person receiving care, their family and carers
- use evidence to support arguments.

There are many reasons why using evidence-based practice in nursing is important; the list below is not exhaustive but is a starting point:

- establishes justifiable, defensible reasons for nursing actions
- ensures patient safety
- increases cost-effective practice
- enhances clinical effectiveness
- is a basis for assuring quality care delivery (clinical governance)
- improves the patient's experience
- provides evidence of what does not work
- provides evidence to support resource allocation
- supports managing risk
- encourages academic and professional development.

(Heaslip and Lindsay, 2018)

RECAP

- Clinical nursing procedures are no longer based on custom and tradition but on evidence – this is known as evidence-based practice.
- The NMC and RCN both emphasise the need for evidence-based practice (EBP), and EBP is a constant theme of the NMC *Future Nurse* standards.

>> Carrying out evidence-based practice

As noted in the introduction to this chapter, several authors, such as Parahoo (2014), Williamson *et al.* (2008) and Sackett *et al.* (2000), suggest a sequence of events has to take place before information can be considered 'evidence-based'. This is summarised in *Figure 7.3*.

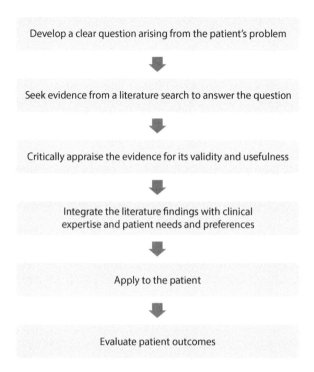

Develop a clear question arising from the patient's problem

Seek evidence from a literature search to answer the question

Critically appraise the evidence for its validity and usefulness

Integrate the literature findings with clinical expertise and patient needs and preferences

Apply to the patient

Evaluate patient outcomes

Figure 7.3: *The sequence of evidence-based practice.*

What is evidence?

In the past, supporters of evidence-based practice have focused on research derived from quantitative methods (data collected in the form of numbers and analysed statistically), as they were deemed the only studies worth considering. There was little or no recognition of research gathered by qualitative means (data collected in the form of words, with a focus on experience and feelings) (Ingersoll, 2000). Dougherty and Lister (2015) believe this is worrying when, within nursing,

>> Evidence is increasingly recognised as coming from many different sources.

qualitative research is the prevalent design used. However, this is changing as increasingly evidence is recognised as coming from many different areas (as shown in *Figure 7.1*) with changing research methodologies including the use of mixed methods (using both quantitative and qualitative data) and the use of non-research evidence, such as audits and narratives of patients' experiences.

Credibility is key in evidence-based practice but there is little consensus about how evidence is assessed before it is used to inform practice, mainly because making such judgements about evidence is complex and difficult to achieve (Dougherty and Lister, 2015). In some instances government bodies have developed nationally accepted guidelines as a result of expert researchers undertaking research trials – examples of these are the NICE (National Institute for Health and Care Excellence) guidelines and National Service Frameworks (NSFs), which were developed to achieve consistent clinical standards across the NHS.

In other instances, hospitals have created their own nursing guidelines, where procedures are regularly reviewed and updated. An example of this is the Royal Marsden Hospital's *Manual of Clinical Nursing Procedures* (Dougherty and Lister, 2015). These are then published, thereby enabling other healthcare professionals and patients to benefit from the work.

ACTIVITY 7.1

Choose one aspect of nursing care. List the sources of evidence needed to ensure the delivery of evidence-based practice to deliver high quality and safe nursing care.

Critical awareness

Society's healthcare needs and expectations are rapidly changing, which requires nurses to have an understanding of not only anatomy and pathophysiology but also sociology and psychology. They need to keep their knowledge up to date if they are to provide the best possible care to patients based on the best available evidence which they need to be able to critically review (NMC, 2018a). Equally, nurses need to challenge everyday practices to ensure they are safe for use with patients, as nurses are their patients'/service users' advocate (NMC, 2018a). A major part of keeping care up to date is reviewing or evaluating literature on a subject. Evaluating research sounds rather daunting for the inexperienced but it can be broken down into a number of simple steps.

First, all research needs to be reliable (truthful) and valid (transferable), but not all research is necessarily relevant or applicable (Heaslip and Lindsay, 2018). Evidence sought needs to be linked directly to nurses' practice and to inform that practice, thereby making it relevant and applicable. Not all research is generalisable (applicable to other settings); an example of this is a project where the use of ordinary tap water for wound cleansing was advocated. However, the study was carried out in a developed country where water is purified – in some countries the water is not purified and may be contaminated, so using tap water in these areas would be unsafe.

Secondly, nurses need to be critical and questioning of the evidence they seek to use to inform their practice, as it is important for them to decide the value or worth of a piece of research, given the purposes for which it is intended. Aveyard and Sharp (2013, p. 111) explain that this involves not just accepting what is written at face value but being able to "interpret what is read", be "selective and critical" and use "best available evidence".

Therefore, thirdly, nurses need to know how to evaluate a research article (Aveyard and Sharp, 2013). As a nurse you are individually accountable (NMC, 2018a), so you need to decide on the reliability and validity of the research. In order to do this it is necessary to develop the skills to evaluate the research evidence in a critical way. Below is guidance for evaluating research articles. This guidance is comprehensive, but you may not be able to address all the points – it depends on the focus of the research article.

The article

The title – is it informative, interesting and to the point? In other words, does it address the question that you want answered?

The authors – what do you know about the authors? Do they have a vested interest in the conclusions of the study?

The abstract – does it summarise the main points of the study adequately and accurately? Be careful, as sometimes abstracts promise more than that which is written in the rest of the paper.

Introduction – is the problem or purpose of the study clearly stated?

The questions – are they stated clearly and concisely? Do they follow logically from the problems? Are they worth answering? Are they answerable?

The literature – is the background information adequate? Does the author appear to know their subject? Do they appraise related research and authoritative statements? Or have they strung together citations and quotes which support their proposal without consideration of antagonistic arguments? Are specific theories used in order to put the study and potentially the findings into context? Does this theory seem relevant?

Relevance – is the study placed in the context of current professional knowledge? What is the potential contribution of the study to practice?

Aims – are the aims stated clearly, concisely and precisely? Are they logically related to the original question(s)? How were they formulated; for example, does evidence from the literature support intuition, instinct and experience? If treatment is being investigated, are the aims related to efficacy and safety?

Methodology

Design – is the study descriptive or experimental? Is it described adequately? Does the chosen design seem appropriate to you? A hypothesis or set of hypotheses is necessary for an experimental design. Does it follow logically from the original problem and theories?

Assumptions – are any assumptions being made? Is their use explained? Are they justifiable and appropriate? Was a pilot study completed, i.e. was a questionnaire or special report pre-tested for validity and reliability? Were modifications made? What were they and why were they made?

Ethical considerations – has the author considered the ethics of the method? Is the proposed method ethically acceptable? For example, will all service users receive the treatment/intervention they need rather than the treatment needed for the study? Will a control group be required to receive a bogus or dummy treatment of dubious efficacy?

Participants – how were people selected? Are individuals allocated to alternative treatment/intervention groups? Is this ethical? Is there an account of how each person was chosen? Were specific criteria used to include people in the study, or exclude them from it? Are these criteria clearly stated? Is the reasoning behind them apparent and sensible?

Samples – was a specific size of sample chosen (for example, for statistical purposes)? Does it seem adequate to provide sustainable results? If the author aims to make general comments about a population on the basis of the findings, who forms this population? Is the sample representative of this population?

Data collection – is the method described adequately? Could you replicate it from the description? Are the reasons for the choice of method stated? If special report forms, assessment forms, questionnaires or interview schedules have been used, are copies provided with the paper or is an address given for copies?

Findings

Analysis – is the method of analysis understandable? Have statistical tests been used? Are reasons for choice given which explain their appropriateness? Do you understand and accept the explanation?

Results – are results intelligible enough for you to interpret them and draw your own conclusions? Are they relevant to the stated problem? Does your background knowledge and common sense indicate that they are realistic and feasible? Is 'raw' data given, or only proportions, percentages, etc., after manipulation? Are histograms, pie charts and other graphic representations explained? Are the tables helpful? If results are based on responses to a questionnaire or interview schedule, what is the response rate? Are statistical results included? Are they meaningful? Is the statistical probability of results by chance included? Is it appropriate?

Discussion – are the results interpreted in relation to the original questions? Are the original questions answered? Have the aims been fulfilled? Does the author discuss any weaknesses in the methodology and factors which may have affected validity or reliability? For example, should sample selection be discussed? If criteria of inclusion and exclusion need clarification, is the explanation acceptable? Should the advantages and disadvantages of the method of data collection be discussed? Are they? Have you noticed anything that was omitted? Has the author referred to it or ignored it? Have the findings been related to the existing body of knowledge and relevant theory? Are the clinical implications discussed? Was the project funded? By whom? Might the results be biased because of the interests of the financing body?

Conclusions – are the author's conclusions logical, valid and reliable according to the data and the findings presented?

Recommendations – are the recommendations self-evident from the reported results? Could you attempt to implement them, and should you? Is this study an end in itself, or does it suggest further research?

References – is the length of the list more impressive than its quality? Are any references conspicuous by their absence?

There are also tools to evaluate research readily accessible, such as the Critical Appraisal Skills Programme (CASP) tools and checklists and the Understanding Health Research appraisal tool. These are available online – see the *Useful websites* at the end of the chapter and *Activity 7.2.*

RECAP

- Evidence can come from different sources and via different methods, including quantitative, qualitative and mixed methods. Evidence may also come from non-research sources such as clinical audits and patient experiences.
- Nurses must be critical and questioning of evidence, including being able to evaluate research articles.

ACTIVITY 7.2

Find a research article in any nursing journal relating to your chosen aspect of nursing care. Review this article using the suggested guidance above or consider using a formal tool or checklist (CASP, available at www.casp-uk.net/appraising-the-evidence or Understanding Health Research, available at www.understandinghealthresearch.org).

» Clinical effectiveness and evidence-based practice

The term 'evidence-based practice' is often linked with clinical effectiveness. Williamson *et al.* (2008) believe clinical effectiveness is concerned with using treatments or care that have been shown to work, and it is important that what nurses do is effective because "the NHS is a publicly funded service and it would be financially wasteful, pointless and immoral ... to be using particular clinical interventions if they were not known to be effective" (Williamson *et al.*, 2008, p. 82).

The link between evidence-based practice and clinical effectiveness is identified within the Department of Health's definition, as cited by the RCN (1996, p. 1) where it is concerned with "applying the best available knowledge, derived from research, clinical expertise and patient preferences, to achieve optimum processes and outcomes of care for patients" – a definition not dissimilar to the definition of evidence-based practice.

Clinical effectiveness is also linked to clinical governance (see also *Chapter 6*) which was introduced by the Department of Health in 1998 to ensure that care provided is of high quality and has effective outcomes. Indeed, all four countries of the UK have identified safe and effective care as part of their individual health strategies (Welsh Government, 2012; Department of Health, Social Services and Public Safety, 2011; Scottish Government, 2010). This can only be achieved by using current evidence to provide patient care in clinical practice.

» Implementing evidence-based practice

As discussed in this chapter, it is imperative for every nursing student and registered nurse to understand and use evidence-based practice to provide clinically effective and safe patient care. However, Dougherty and Lister (2015) point out that, on the whole, delivering evidence-based care can be demanding and needs determination and time. Craig and Smyth (2012) summarise the findings of the review by Kajermo *et al.* (2010) of 53 studies that used the Barriers Scale (Funk *et al.*, 1991). They state that "the barriers most consistently highly ranked featured the inaccessibility of evidence (whether due to incomprehensible statistics, poorly synthesised or publicised findings), nurses' research skill deficits and lack of authority, resources and support to support change" (ibid., p. 292). Thus, obstacles can include:
- the language of evidence
- poor skills in evaluating evidence
- organisational factors such as workload and staffing

- the inability to change
- the possibility that there is no evidence available
- the possibility that the evidence is not transferable from one clinical setting to another.

Nevertheless, despite these challenges it remains incumbent on nurses to use current best evidence when providing information and care and to be able to justify this (NMC, 2018b, p. 7); thus, delivering evidence-based practice is every nurse's role. Nurses need to be motivated to find strategies to overcome these barriers within their day-to-day practice. This includes individual nurses developing the skills to search for the evidence and being able to critically appraise/evaluate it, as well as developing an understanding of how to effect change. As Gerrish and Lathlean (2015, p. 542) emphasise, "commitment is needed from individual nurses together with support from colleagues within the multidisciplinary team and from managers".

>> Delivering evidence-based practice is every nurse's role.

Finally, it is important to remember that within the delivery of evidence-based nursing practice, person-centred care is given. Accordingly, the patient/service user is a partner in their care, so the assessment of their clinical situation and their preferences needs to be taken into account.

ACTIVITY 7.3

In *Activity 7.1*, you were asked to choose one aspect of nursing care and list the sources of evidence needed to ensure the delivery of evidence-based practice to deliver high quality and safe nursing care. Read the sources of evidence you have found and reflect on what you have observed in practice. Is there a difference? If so, what would you do about it? Consider the NMC (2018a) *Code: professional standards of practice and behaviour for nurses, midwives and nursing associates* in your reflection.

CHAPTER SUMMARY

- All care given should be based on evidence-based practice and be non-discriminatory.
- The care must be appropriate for the individual patient/service user (person-centred).
- Evidence-based practice is often linked with clinical effectiveness, clinical governance, patient safety and health outcomes.

Further information

This chapter does not attempt to discuss research methodologies, nor how to seek out literature – there are many textbooks that can help you with that. An example is Vanessa Heaslip and Bruce Lindsay's 2018 book, *Research and Evidence-Based Practice: for nursing, health and social care students* (Lantern Publishing).

References

Aveyard, H. and Sharp, P. (2013) *A Beginner's Guide to Evidence Based Practice in Health and Social Care*, 2nd edition. Maidenhead: Open University Press.

Bury, T. and Mead, J. (1998) *Evidence Based Health Care: a practical guide for therapists.* Oxford: Butterworth-Heinemann.

Craig, J. and Smyth, R. (2012) *The Evidence-based Practice Manual for Nurses,* 3rd edition. Edinburgh: Churchill Livingstone.

Cullum, N., Ciliska, D., Haynes, R. and Marks, S. (eds) (2008) *Evidence-based Nursing: an introduction.* Oxford: Blackwell.

Cummings, J. and Bennett, V. for the Department of Health (2012) *Compassion in Practice: nursing, midwifery and care staff – our vision and strategy.* Available at: www.england.nhs.uk/wp-content/uploads/2012/12/compassion-in-practice.pdf (accessed 3 April 2019)

Department of Health, Social Services and Public Safety (2011) *Quality 2020: a 10 year strategy to protect and improve quality in health and social care in Northern Ireland.* Belfast: DHSSPS.

Dougherty, L. and Lister, S. (2015) *The Royal Marsden Hospital Manual of Clinical Nursing Procedures,* 9th edition. Chichester: Wiley-Blackwell.

Funk, S., Champagne, M., Wiese, R. and Tornquist, E. (1991) BARRIERS: the barriers to research utilization scale. *Applied Nursing Research,* 4(1): 39–45. Available at: http://doi:10.1016/S0897-1897(05)80052-7 (accessed 9 April 2019)

Gerrish, K. and Lathlean, J. (eds) (2015) *The Research Process in Nursing,* 7th edition. Oxford: Wiley-Blackwell.

Heaslip, V. and Lindsay, B. (2018) *Research and Evidence-Based Practice: for nursing, health and social care students.* Banbury: Lantern Publishing Ltd.

Ingersoll, G. (2000) Evidence-based nursing: what it is and what it isn't. *Nursing Outlook,* 48(4): 151–2.

Kajermo, K., Boström, A-M., Thompson, D., Hutchinson, A. Estabrooks, C. and Wallin, L. (2010) The BARRIERS scale – the barriers to research utilization scale: a systematic review. *Implementation Science,* 5: 32. Available at: https//doi.org/10.1186/1748-5908-5-32 (accessed 9 April 2019)

McClarey, M. and Duff, L. (1997) Clinical effectiveness and evidence-based practice. *Nursing Standard,* 11(52): 33–7.

NHS England (2015) *NHS Constitution for England.* Available at: www.gov.uk/government/publications/the-nhs-constitution-for-england (accessed 9 April 2019)

Nursing and Midwifery Council (2018a) *The Code: professional standards of practice and behaviour for nurses, midwives and nursing associates.* London: NMC.

Nursing and Midwifery Council (2018b) *Future Nurse: standards of proficiency for registered nurses.* London: NMC.

Parahoo, K. (2014) *Nursing Research: principles, process and issues.* Basingstoke: Palgrave Macmillan.

Royal College of Nursing (1996) *Clinical Effectiveness.* London: RCN.

Rycroft-Malone, J., Seers, K., Titchen, A., Harvey, G., Kitson, A. & McCormack, B. (2004) What counts as evidence in evidence-based practice? *Journal of Advanced Nursing,* 47(1): 81–90.

Sackett, D., Rosenberg, W., Gray, J., Haynes, R. & Richardson, W. (1996) Evidence based medicine: what it is and what it isn't. *British Medical Journal*, **312**: 71–2.

Sackett, D., Straus, S., Richardson, W., Rosenberg, W. & Haynes, R. (2000) *Evidence-Based Medicine. how to practice and teach EBM*, 2nd edition. London: Churchill Livingstone.

Scottish Government (2010) *The Healthcare Quality Strategy for NHS Scotland*. Edinburgh: Scottish Government.

Welsh Government (2012) *Achieving Excellence: the quality delivery plan for the NHS in Wales*. Cardiff: Welsh Government.

Williamson, G., Jenkinson, T. and Proctor-Childs, T. (2008) *Nursing in Contemporary Healthcare Practice*. Exeter: Learning Matters.

Useful websites

https://casp-uk.net/casp-tools-checklists/ (accessed 2 May 2019)
www.nice.org.uk (accessed 9 April 2019)
www.thecochranelibrary.com (accessed 9 April 2019)
www.understandinghealthresearch.org (accessed 9 April 2019)

PROFESSIONAL ROLES IN HEALTHCARE

The aim of this chapter is to provide a brief overview of interprofessional practice and outline some career opportunities after graduation.

LEARNING OUTCOMES

On completion of this chapter you should be able to:
- understand the concept and context of interprofessional practice
- recognise some of the benefits and challenges of interprofessional practice
- appreciate why nurses' roles change
- be aware of some of the career options that are open to you as a registered nurse

» Introduction to interprofessional practice

Since the beginnings of the NHS in 1948, the provision of healthcare in the UK has undergone a variety of changes in terms of organisational restructuring, managerial and economic change. Many of these changes have resulted in the fragmentation of health and social care services since the 1990s and particularly since the implementation of the Community Care Act. This has meant that healthcare is delivered by the NHS and social care is provided by Local Authorities. Healthcare and social care have different funding arrangements from central government and they are both subject to government funding policies that are liable to change. In addition, some health and social care is provided by the voluntary sector or non-government organisations, which are independently self-financing, and also by the private sector. This means that the care you provide as a nurse involves working in a multidisciplinary or interprofessional team which will comprise many different health and social care professionals who have their own individual professional cultures and forms of accountability.

» The care you provide as a nurse will involve working in a team of many different health and social care professionals.

The NMC *Code* (2018a) explicitly states that a nurse must work cooperatively. The expectation is that a nurse will "play an active and equal role in the inter-disciplinary team, collaborating and communicating effectively with a range of colleagues" (NMC, 2018b, p. 19). This includes having an understanding of the roles and scope of practice of not only all the members of the nursing team but also the interdisciplinary team.

As a nurse you are an equal member of an interdisciplinary team and will be required to have the ability to communicate effectively both face to face and via digital technologies, including with agencies external to your organisation (see also *Chapter 2*), as well as the ability to be assertive and challenge "and provide constructive feedback about care delivered by others in the team" (ibid., Clause 5.9). Furthermore, it is necessary that you understand the wider context of working in teams; that is, "the principles of human factors, environmental factors and strength-based approaches when working in teams" (ibid., Clause 5.2).

» Definitions

There are a number of terms associated with or used in the context of interprofessional practice which can be confusing. The following are those you are most likely to come into contact with:

- **Uni-disciplinary** – professional groups working independently of each other.
- **Partnership** – "is a state of relationships, at organisational, group, professional or inter-professional level to be achieved, maintained and reviewed" (Whittington, 2003, cited by Quinney and Hafford-Letchfield, 2009, p. 16).
- **Collaboration** – "is an active process of partnership in action" (ibid., p. 16).
- **Multiprofessional/multidisciplinary** – two or more practitioner groups, either from the same professional background, or from different disciplines who work side by side (Glasby and Dickinson, 2014, p. 149); for example, nurses and doctors.
- **Inter-agency/multi-agency** – practitioners from two or more organisations/ agencies who work together (Glasby and Dickinson, 2014, p. 149); for example, NHS and Social Care.
- **Intraprofessional/intradisciplinary** – a professional group that is further divided into smaller sections, each with its own specific area of specialism, such as, for example, nursing – adult, paediatric, mental health, health visiting, district nursing. Intersecting lines of communication and collaboration exist between these professional specialisms.
- **Interprofessional/interdisciplinary** – intersecting lines of communication and collaboration between different professions and agencies (for example, health and social care, nursing and allied health professionals); the groups are more

integrated and all modify their efforts to take account of other team members' contributions (Leathard, 2003; Day, 2013; ACCP, 2009).

- **Integrated care** – "care that is person-centred and co-ordinated within healthcare settings, across mental and physical health and across health and social care" (UK Government, 2015).

ACTIVITY 8.1

Consider each of the definitions above and try to relate it to any previous experience you may have had in a care/work environment. Note down the benefits and challenges of working within an interprofessional team.

>> Interprofessional working

A review of the literature (Thomas *et al.*, 2014; Leathard, 2003; Hammick *et al.*, 2009) suggests there is a general consensus, not only in the political arena but also among health and social care professionals, that interprofessional practice can provide many positive benefits to both the practitioners involved and the service users/patients they care for. The identified benefits of such practice include that it:

>> Interprofessional practice can provide many positive benefits to both patients and practitioners.

- allows for streamlining of services (usually driven by government policy)
- provides for a more effective use of staff
- offers increased overall quality of service provision
- provides better use of limited resources (driven by economic factors).

For the practitioners involved, interprofessional practice also:

- increases work satisfaction
- can encourage development of mutual respect, mutual cooperation and empathy between professionals
- should improve communication between different professionals and provide social support, which could potentially prevent stress and burnout
- allows all members of the team to understand each other's roles and recognise areas of overlap within the traditional disciplines
- can encourage a greater understanding of the difference between accountability and responsibility of different team members and what is expected of them (each profession has its own professional code)
- provide a more holistic and person-centred approach to care.

Benefits for service users/patients include:
- continuity and consistency of care within a seamless service
- decrease of ambiguity in the information being given to the patient
- appropriate referral because of the greater understanding of other professionals' roles
- care being based on a holistic perspective with the best-placed professionals providing person-centred care.

(Miller *et al.*, 2001)

According to Keeping (2014, pp. 23–8) for the benefits of interprofessional practice to be fully maximised, not only does it require complex interactions between practitioners, but also knowledge and attitudes:
- knowledge of professional roles
- knowledge of policy developments
- willing participation
- open and honest communication
- trust and mutual respect
- personal and professional confidence
- teamworking skills.

Knowledge of professional roles

As noted above, in order for effective interprofessional practice to take place to benefit the patient/service user, it is essential that each team member has an understanding of the role and professional boundaries of other practitioners they may be working with. This includes understanding your own professional role, identity and boundaries – refer to the NMC *Code* (2018a).

ACTIVITY 8.2

You may already be participating in shared learning with other professional groups; take some time to talk to them about their specific role and function within the care environment.

Knowledge of policy developments

Both health and social care services, in all four UK nations, are changing as the result of their respective varying political philosophies, demographic changes and economic factors. Government policies impact on the way in which daily care is, and will be, delivered. It is therefore necessary that all health and social care practitioners, including nurses, are aware of their current national political drivers and policies, as well as local policies.

Willing participation

High levels of motivation and willingness of the participants are pivotal to the effectiveness of any interprofessional collaboration. Maintaining such motivation and willingness, even if unsatisfactory experiences of interprofessional practice are encountered, is very important (Molyneux, 2001; Pollard, 2009).

Personal and professional confidence

Writers such as Leathard (2003) suggest that the most basic requirement for interprofessional collaboration must be the individual's own professional competence. They argue that until the practitioner feels confident that they are an expert in their own field, and are regarded as such by their peers, they are unlikely to feel sufficiently secure to engage fully in sharing practice with others outside their own professional arena. Personal levels of confidence within the practice area will increase as you progress through your student nurse programme and after you qualify.

Open and honest communication

Open and honest communication is linked very closely to internal feelings associated with an individual's level of confidence. It also involves the need for the participants to set aside any assumptions and judgements they may have about other professions involved in the collaborative practice (Interprofessional Education Collaborative Panel, 2011).

Trust and mutual respect

Trust can be viewed as a vital characteristic of collaboration, and another component that develops over time through repeated positive interprofessional experiences, both in the classroom and in practice. According to Keeping (2014), trust is based on mutual respect which develops when all participants feel valued, both individually and organisationally.

Teamworking skills

According to Pett (2017, pp. 93–6), essential skills for effective teamworking include "being authentic and self-aware". Reflection is an important skill in relation to developing self-awareness (see also *Chapter 9*). In addition, "positive relationships and good communication" (see also *Chapter 2*) are needed (Keeping, 2014, p. 28). The ability to be assertive and open to feedback, as well as to resolve conflicts, are also necessary skills (NMC, 2018b).

Furthermore, for interprofessional working to be effective, supportive management/organisational structures are required. Keeping (2014) suggests management strategies that can be put in place are:

- reflection through clinical supervision (this could be individual or group)
- learning together within interprofessional education and training
- team development
- profession-specific meetings to maintain professional identities
- establishing guidelines relating to the parameters within which individual professions work.

In addition, when delivering person-centred care as part of the team, the role of lay carers is important. These are non-professional carers, e.g. family or friends, who provide help and assistance (Peate and Wild, 2018). Taking on a caring role can happen at any time and as a child or an adult. It is estimated that there are 6.5 million carers in the UK (CarersUK, 2015). Each of the four nations of the UK has legislation in place relating to carers: the Carers Act (2014) for England, the Social Services and Well-being (Wales) Act 2014, Carers (Scotland) Act (2016) and Carers and Direct Payments Act (Northern Ireland) (2002). These Acts ensure that carers' needs are assessed regardless of their financial situation or level of need (Peate and Wild, 2018). Specific legislation such as the Children and Families Act (2014) for England aims to ensure that young carers have the right to an assessment and to have any identified needs met. Lay carers have an important role in supporting the care provided and are a crucial source of information about the patient/service user. Involving them in the care can enhance the quality of care given.

≫ Challenges to successful interprofessional working

Despite the recognised benefits there are still some difficulties with, and barriers to, effective and widespread interprofessional practice, particularly within health and social care. These include:

- organisational issues – between health and social services, such as, for example, disparity of boundaries (both geographical and professional) and centres of control
- operational matters – different budgetary and planning sequences and procedures
- monetary factors – including different funding structures and sources of financial resources
- status and validity – social care is directed through democratically elected and appointed agencies, i.e. local authorities, whereas healthcare is directed by policy from central government and the Department of Health through the NHS

- professional issues – these are numerous and include:
    - problems associated with differing ideologies, values and language
    - conflicting views about users
    - separate training backgrounds
    - differing organisational boundaries and professional loyalties
    - inequalities in status and pay
    - lack of clarity about roles, historical prejudices and power relationships
    - professional defence of professions and an unwillingness to dilute them in any way (professional protectionism)
    - differences between specialisms, expertise and skills – this can include medical practitioners (and can occur intraprofessionally as well as interprofessionally).

(Leathard, 2003; Day, 2013)

However, ongoing government policy, legislation and directives and the inclusion of interprofessional education and training for health and social care professionals all seek to lessen the impact of the above factors. Indeed, the current emphasis within health and social care is the move towards integrated care in order to provide more responsive, seamless person-centred care. It is intended that this will lead to better planning and use of resources which will be cost-effective, as well as increasing the involvement of the patient/service user in their care provision (UK Government, 2015). The delivery of this type of care includes the development of generic workers who will have the competencies to work across both the health and social care sectors.

RECAP

- Interprofessional working can provide benefits to practitioners and patients/ service users, but it requires complex interactions between professionals and particular knowledge and attitudes.
- There are some barriers to interprofessional working that health and social care policy seeks to overcome.

FURTHER READING
Discussion of a range of issues associated with interprofessional practice can be found both online and through journals such as the *Journal of Interprofessional Care*, which promotes collaboration in education, practice and research for health and social care, and the *Journal of Research in Interprofessional Practice and Education*, which disseminates theoretical perspectives, methodologies and evidence-based knowledge to inform interprofessional practice.

>> Changing roles in nursing

Why the need for change?

As noted in *Chapter 7*, society and people's health needs are changing rapidly, with more people living longer and living with one or more long-term condition. There is also a need to address health inequalities (see also *Chapter 11*). Furthermore, with national policy and economic changes, the fast-changing pace of technology and the ways it can be used in healthcare, together with the advances in research in understanding diseases

>> Nurses need to develop their skills and knowledge continually through lifelong learning.

and the development of new and innovative treatments and care plans, nurses will need to adapt and continually develop their skills and knowledge through education and lifelong learning.

The International Council of Nurses (ICN) (2010) offers a definition of nursing that encompasses the vast arena of care that nurses deliver. While it is accepted that not all nurses are involved in all the aspects of nursing described at any one time, nurses still need to be flexible, adaptable, innovative and resilient in order to respond to the changing needs and perceptions of their patients. In addition, a market-driven health service and ever-changing reforms require their role to be continuously evolving and changing.

THE ICN DEFINITION OF NURSING

"Nursing encompasses autonomous and collaborative care of individuals of all ages, families, groups and communities, sick or well and in all settings. Nursing includes the promotion of health, prevention of illness, and the care of ill, disabled and dying people. Advocacy, promotion of a safe environment, research, participation in shaping health policy and in patient and health systems management, and education are also key nursing roles" (ICN, 2010).

Policy context

Probably the most profound impact on a nurse's work life in recent years has been the introduction of the *NHS Plan* (Department of Health, 2000). This has since been superseded by other government initiatives, but at the time, the *Plan* represented the biggest change to healthcare in England since the NHS was formed in 1948. Along with setting out reform of the NHS, it included a section on the roles nurses should undertake and "encouraged nurses and other staff to extend their roles".

In 2014, the NHS *Five Year Forward View* plan was published, which identifies how the healthcare system needs to change. Within this plan is an emphasis on prevention of ill health (see also *Chapter 11*), the patient/service user having more control over their care, and the move towards care being giving more locally, with a focus on provision in the community rather than hospital. It also anticipates a closer working relationship between general practitioners (GPs) and hospitals as well as services provided in specialist centres which will be organised in such a way to meet the needs of patients/service users (NHS, 2014). New models of care delivery are being introduced:

- Multispecialty community provider – GPs will be able to unite with nurses and other community health services, hospital specialists and potentially even with mental health and social care in order to construct "integrated out-of-hospital care" (ibid., p. 4)
- Primary and acute care systems – integration of hospital and primary care (community) providers
- Urgent and emergency care – redesigned at local level.

The advancement of this plan was reviewed in 2017, and it suggested that progress has been made. The aim now is to speed up the process of redesigning local services, improve access to Accident and Emergency, improve cancer and mental health services and access to GPs (NHS, 2017).

Many of the changes in the health service today, which include the role of the nurse, have been driven not only by policy and economic changes but also by patients. Patient perceptions and expectations of their healthcare have risen as information on medical and nursing roles has been made more accessible (particularly via the internet) and transparent. However, the changing roles of other healthcare professionals (notably changes resulting from the European Working Time Directive which mean that, with some exceptions and exemptions, someone cannot legally work more than 48 hours per week) have also had an impact on the nurse's role, and in some instances have led to the creation of brand new roles for nurses.

>> Nursing in the 21st century in the UK

The NMC (2018b) document *Future Nurse: standards of proficiency for registered nurses* states that in the 21st century:

- *"Registered nurses play a vital role in providing, leading and coordinating care that is compassionate, evidence-based and person-centred.*
- *They are accountable for their own actions and must be able to work autonomously, or as an equal partner with a range of other professionals, and in interdisciplinary teams.*

- *In order to respond to the impact and demands of professional nursing practice, they must be emotionally intelligent and resilient individuals, who are able to manage their own personal health and wellbeing, and know when and how to access support.*
- *Registered nurses make an important contribution to the promotion of health, health protection and the prevention of ill health.*
- *They do this by empowering people, communities and populations to exercise choice, take control of their own health decisions and behaviours, and by supporting people to manage their own care where possible.*
- *Registered nurses provide leadership in the delivery of care for people of all ages and from different backgrounds, cultures and beliefs.*
- *They provide nursing care for people who have complex mental, physical, cognitive and behavioural care needs, those living with dementia, the elderly, and for people at the end of their life.*
- *They must be able to care for people in their own home, in the community or hospital or in any healthcare settings where their needs are supported and managed.*
- *They work in the context of continual change, challenging environments, different models of care delivery, shifting demographics, innovation, and rapidly evolving technologies.*
- *Increasing integration of health and social care services will require registered nurses to negotiate boundaries and play a proactive role in interdisciplinary teams.*
- *The confidence and ability to think critically, apply knowledge and skills, and provide expert, evidence-based, direct nursing care therefore lies at the centre of all registered nursing practice."*

(NMC, 2018b, p. 3)

RECAP

- Nursing roles change over time because of changes in people's healthcare needs, in response to government policy, and as a result of developments in technology and patients' expectations.
- The NMC's 2018 document *Future Nurse* sets out the role of the nurse in the 21st century and reflects what the public can expect nurses to know and be able to do in order to deliver safe, compassionate and effective nursing care.

» Careers in nursing

Nurses work in many differing health and social care areas, both within hospitals and the community, and many develop expertise in specific disease areas. This leads to a variety of roles that can be pursued within nursing. Some of these roles which nurses currently undertake are considered below. This is not an exhaustive list, but highlights the concept of nurses working beyond their initial registration.

District nurse

A district nurse must be a qualified nurse (in either adult, child, mental health or learning disabilities) and have undertaken a specialist practitioner programme (minimum first-degree level, i.e. level 6). These programmes are normally no less than one academic year (32 weeks) full-time or part-time equivalent (although they may be completed in a shorter period of time where credit is given for prior learning). Community staff nurses, who are registered nurses, can be funded onto the specialist programme via their individual employer.

District nurses are an integral part of the primary healthcare team. They provide nursing care to patients during periods of illness/incapacity in non-hospital settings. This is usually in the patient's own home but can also be in residential care homes, health centres or GP surgeries. Patients may be of any age and include those who are housebound, elderly, terminally ill, disabled and those recently discharged from hospital.

The district nurse's work is diverse but their main activities include:
- accepting referrals from other professionals and agencies such as, for example, hospitals and GPs
- assessing, planning and managing the care of patients within their caseload
- establishing links with patients' families and carers and, where appropriate, working with them to develop their skills in caring for the patient
- working both intra- and interprofessionally with a range of other professionals and agencies within the NHS, social care, independent and voluntary sector
- playing a fundamental role in promoting healthy lifestyles and health education/teaching
- prescribing from an identified list
- being accountable for the care they deliver.
               (See www.nmc.org.uk; www.rcn.org.uk; www.healthcareers.nhs.uk)

Health visitor

A health visitor must have a degree in either adult or children's nursing or be a registered midwife. They must also have undertaken an approved specialist community public health nursing (health visiting) programme (SCPHN/HV). The programmes normally comprise 45 weeks' study to be completed within a 156-week period (part-time study should be completed within 208 weeks). Accreditation of prior learning can be applied to a maximum of one-third of an

SCPHN/HV programme. Course funding is usually through the individual's employer, although a few people may fund themselves.

Health visitors are usually part of the primary healthcare team and their role involves working in clinics and doctors' surgeries, as well as visiting people in their own homes. Health visitors undertake a range of work including:

- leading and delivering child and family health services (pregnancy through to five years)
- providing ongoing additional services for vulnerable children and families
- contributing to multidisciplinary services in safeguarding and protecting children
- focusing on the prevention and early detection of ill health and the promotion of healthy lifestyles
- participating in the design, implementation and evaluation of public health programmes.

(See www.nmc.org.uk; www.rcn.org.uk; www.healthcareers.nhs.uk)

School nurse

To become a school nurse, you need to be a registered nurse (adult, child, mental health or learning disabilities) or midwife and undertake an approved Specialist Community Public Health Nursing (SCPHN) programme. No minimum post-registration experience is required. This programme is degree level and normally takes one year; it consists of 45 weeks' study to be completed within a 156-week period (part-time study should be completed within 208 weeks). Accreditation of prior learning can be applied to a maximum of one-third of an SCPHN programme. Course funding is usually through employer sponsorship. School nurses work closely with GPs, the health and social care workforce and health visitors and may be employed by local councils, the NHS or by individual schools. They:

- carry out health assessments
- make home visits to families in need
- provide health education and advice, and signpost to other sources of information
- provide immunisation clinics
- advise and support schools with their public health agendas, e.g. healthy eating advice, smoking cessation programmes
- support safeguarding and service coordination
- give advice on childhood diseases.

(See www.healthcareers.nhs.uk/explore-roles/public-health/roles-public-health/school-nurse)

General practice nurse

General practice nurses work in GP surgeries as part of the primary healthcare team and are employed by GPs. You must be a registered nurse (adult, child, mental health or learning disabilities). Training and development are available; for example, in managing long-term conditions. There are degree and master's level programmes in community specialist practice (practice nursing), which normally take one year full-time equivalent. This can lead to becoming a nurse practitioner. Normally you need to be sponsored for these programmes by your employer. In the first instance, contact a GP surgery for more information about the role and possible training opportunities.

The age range of patients that are seen by general practice nurses varies from babies to end-of-life within individually arranged appointments. They may also hold specific clinics, e.g. for vaccinations and immunisations or patients with asthma.

General practice nurses can be involved in:
- obtaining blood samples
- electrocardiograms (ECGs)
- minor and complex wound management, including leg ulcers
- travel health advice and vaccinations
- child immunisations and advice
- family planning and women's health, including cervical smears
- men's health screening
- sexual health services
- smoking cessation.

(See www.healthcareers.nhs.uk/explore-roles/nursing/roles-nursing/general-practice-nurse)

Advanced nursing practice

You may hear the term 'advanced nurse practitioner'. As you can see from the Royal College of Nursing's definition of advanced practice below, it is not a specific role.

"Advanced practice is a level of practice, rather than a type of practice. Advanced Nurse Practitioners are educated at Master's Level in clinical practice and have been assessed as competent in practice using their expert clinical knowledge and skills. They have the freedom and authority to act, making autonomous decisions in the assessment, diagnosis and treatment of patients"

(RCN, 2018b, p. 4)

The criteria for a nurse to be working at this level would be that they have:
- a relevant master's degree
- non-medical prescribing qualification
- experience and expertise mapped against the four pillars of advanced nursing practice [which are clinical, management and leadership, education and research]
- a job plan that demonstrates current advanced level practice verified by a senior nurse/employer
- a clinical reference verifying the applicant's clinical competence
- evidence of continued professional development related to advanced nursing practice over the previous three years
- a qualification in Health Assessment.

(RCN, 2018b, p. 5)

(See www.rcn.org.uk/professional-development/professional-services/credentialing)

Nurse consultant

The role of nurse consultant also formed part of the national nursing strategy of 1999 (Department of Health, 1999a). Nurse consultants are very experienced registered nurses, who will specialise in a particular field of healthcare and help to provide patients with services that are fast and convenient. Each consultant role will be very different, depending on the needs of the employer, but nurses working at this level are amongst the highest paid of their professions. There will be an expectation to have a master's degree to fulfil this role.

Nurse consultants often spend a minimum of 50 per cent of their time working directly with patients, ensuring that people using the NHS continue to benefit from the very best nursing skills. In addition, they are responsible for developing personal practice, being involved in research and evaluation and contributing to education, training and development.

(See www.healthcareers.nhs.uk/explore-roles/nursing/
roles-nursing/adult-nurse/training-and-development-adult-nursing)

Nurse prescriber

Since 1994 some nurses have been able to prescribe medicines for certain groups of patients. In 1999 the *Review of Prescribing, Supply and Administration of Medicines* (Department of Health, 1999b) put forward key principles for the extension of prescribing rights. These

>> Nurse prescribers can only prescribe drugs that are within their area of expertise and level of competence.

principles included the need for appropriate training, regulation and updating, and the need for prescribing to take place within a framework of accountability and competency. The NMC has adopted the Royal Pharmaceutical Society's Competency Framework for All Prescribers. These competencies focus on three areas; the patient, the consultation and the prescribing governance. For a nurse to become a nurse prescriber, they must meet the knowledge requirements and competencies of the Standards for Prescribing Programmes (NMC, 2018d) by attending and successfully completing an NMC-approved programme of study, enabling annotation to their registration with the NMC. A nurse will need one year's post-registration experience before they can undertake a nurse prescribing course.

There are three titles for a nurse or specialist community public health nurse (SCPHN) prescriber:
1. **Community practitioner nurse** or **midwife prescriber:** "this refers to a registered nurse (level 1), midwife or SCPHN (e.g. district nurse, health visitor, school nurse) who has an annotation next to their name on our register confirming that they are qualified to prescribe drugs, medicines and appliances from the *Nurse Prescribers' Formulary for Community Practitioners* in the current edition of the *British National Formulary*" (NMC, 2018d, p. 6).
2. **Nurse** or **midwife independent prescriber:** "this refers to a registered nurse (level 1), midwife or SCPHN who has an annotation next to their name on our register confirming that they may prescribe any medicine for any medical condition within their competence (with the exception of certain controlled drugs)" (NMC, 2018d, p. 7).
3. **Supplementary prescriber:** "this refers to a registered nurse (level 1), midwife or SCPHN who has an annotation next to their name on our register confirming that they are able to work in partnership with an independent prescriber (such as a doctor or dentist) to implement an agreed patient/ client-specific clinical management plan with the patient/client's agreement" (NMC, 2018d, p. 7).

It is important to remember that a nurse prescriber can only prescribe drugs that are within their area of expertise and level of competence, and should only prescribe for children if they have the expertise and competence to do so. Additionally they must comply with current prescribing legislation and are accountable for their practice. Thus, all nurse prescribers must comply with current prescribing legislation within the country they practise in and with local policies and protocols, as well as Royal Pharmaceutical Society recommendations and guidance.

Matrons

In the mid-2000s, the concept of the Modern Matron was introduced to provide strong clinical leadership on wards that was highly visible and accessible to patients (Department of Health, 2003). They are normally senior sisters or charge nurses who lead by example in improving the patient experience and the quality of clinical care, and empowering nurses to take on a greater range of clinical tasks to help improve patient care.

Their ten key responsibilities are:
- leading by example
- making sure patients get quality care
- ensuring staffing is appropriate to patient needs
- empowering nurses to take on a wider range of clinical tasks
- improving hospital cleanliness
- ensuring patients' nutritional needs are met
- improving wards for patients
- making sure patients are treated with respect
- preventing hospital-acquired infection
- resolving problems for patients and their relatives by building closer relationships.

(Department of Health, 2003, p. 4)

The matron role was further expanded in 2005 to the community as part of the 2004 NHS Improvement Plan (NHS, 2004). The community matron role assists in reducing unplanned hospital admissions of patients/service users with long-term conditions.

Nurse educator

There are many teaching roles in nursing. To support learning in practice there are now practice supervisors, practice assessors and academic assessors. The NMC (2018c) publication, *Realising Professionalism: standards for education and training; Part 2: Standards for student supervision and assessment*, details their specific roles and responsibilities.

In addition there are further opportunities open to nurses; usually a Post-graduate Certificate in Healthcare Education (PGCHE) is required, which can lead to further registration with the NMC as a lecturer/practice educator (LPE) or teacher (TCH). The following opportunities are available:
- Practice educator
- Practice education facilitator
- Clinical educator

- Clinical trainer
- Clinical practice lead
- Clinical nurse lead
- Practice development lead
- Nurse educator
- Nurse lecturer

(RCN, 2018a)

As well as the opportunity to obtain a teaching qualification there are extensive opportunities for post-registration study at master's (level 7) and PhD (level 8). Taught professional PhDs as well as research PhDs are available.

If you are interested in pursuing a career in any of these roles or undertaking further educational programmes/courses, then an initial conversation with your personal or professional tutor/academic assessor is a good starting point. Also, remember the nurse's role is always changing, so new opportunities may evolve.

CHAPTER SUMMARY

- There is a general consensus both in the political arena and among care professionals that interprofessional practice is a positive action for both practitioners and service users.
- High levels of motivation and willingness of the participants are pivotal to the effectiveness of any interprofessional collaboration.
- Despite the recognised benefits, there are some difficulties with, and barriers to effective and widespread interprofessional practice, particularly with health and social care.
- There are a number of career opportunities which registered nurses can train for after registration.

References

ACCP (2009) *ACCP White Paper – Inter-professional Education: principles and application. A framework for clinical pharmacy*. Available at: www.accp.com/docs/positions/whitepapers/interprofeduc.pdf (accessed 10 April 2019)

CarersUK (2015) *Facts and Figures*. Available at: www.carersuk.org/news-and-campaigns/press-releases/facts-and-figures (accessed 10 April 2019)

Day, J. (2013) *Interprofessional Working: an essential guide for health and social care professionals*. Andover: Cengage Learning.

Department of Health (1999a) *Making a Difference: strengthening the nursing, midwifery and health visiting contribution to health and health care*. London: DH.

Department of Health (1999b) *Review of Prescribing, Supply and Administration of Medicines*. London: DH.

Department of Health (2000) *The NHS Plan*. London: DH.

Department of Health (2003) *Modern Matrons: improving the patient experience*. London: DH.

Glasby, J. and Dickinson, H. (2014) *Partnership Working in Health and Social Care: what is integrated care and how can we deliver it?* Bristol: Policy Press.

Hammick, M., Freeth, D., Copperman, J. and Goodsman, D. (2009) *Being Interprofessional.* Cambridge: Polity Press.

International Council of Nurses (2010) *Definition of Nursing.* Available at: www.icn.ch/nursing-policy/nursing-definitions (accessed 10 April 2019)

Interprofessional Education Collaborative Panel (2011) *Core Competencies for Interprofessional Collaborative Practice: report of an expert panel.* Washington, DC: Interprofessional Education Collaborative. Available at: https://www.aacom.org/docs/default-source/insideome/ccrpt05-10-11.pdf?sfvrsn=77937f97_2 (accessed 10 May 2019)

Keeping, C. (2014) 'The process required for effective interprofessional working'. In Thomas, J., Pollard, K. and Sellman, D. *Interprofessional Working in Health and Social Care: professional perspectives*, 2ⁿᵈ edition. Basingstoke: Palgrave Macmillan.

Leathard, A. (2003) *Interprofessional Collaboration: from policy to practice in health and social care.* Hove: Routledge.

Miller, C., Freeman, M. and Ross, N. (2001) *Interprofessional Practice in Health and Social Care: challenging the shared learning agenda.* London: Arnold.

Molyneux, J. (2001) Interprofessional teamworking: what makes teams work well? *Journal of Interprofessional Care,* **15(1):** 29–35.

NHS (2004) *NHS Improvement Plan: putting people at the heart of public services.* Available at: http://1nj5ms2lli5hdggbe3mm7ms5.wpengine.netdna-cdn.com/files/2010/03/pnsuk3.pdf (accessed 10 April 2019)

NHS (2014) *Five Year Forward View.* Available at: www.england.nhs.uk/wp-content/uploads/2014/10/5yfv-web.pdf (accessed 10 April 2019)

NHS (2017) *Next Steps on the Five Year Forward View.* Available at: www.england.nhs.uk/wp-content/uploads/2017/03/NEXT-STEPS-ON-THE-NHS-FIVE-YEAR-FORWARD-VIEW.pdf (accessed 10 April 2019)

Nursing and Midwifery Council (2018a) *The Code: professional standards of practice and behaviour for nurses, midwives and nursing associates.* London: NMC.

Nursing and Midwifery Council (2018b) *Future Nurse: standards of proficiency for registered nurses.* London: NMC.

Nursing and Midwifery Council (2018c) *Realising Professionalism: Standards for education and training. Part 2: Standards for student supervision and assessment.* Available at: https://www.nmc.org.uk/Student-supervision-assessment (accessed 10 April 2019)

Nursing and Midwifery Council (2018d) *Realising Professionalism: Standards for education and training. Part 3: Standards for prescribing programmes.* Available at: www.nmc.org.uk/globalassets/sitedocuments/education-standards/programme-standards-prescribing.pdf (accessed 10 April 2019)

Peate, I. and Wild, K. (eds) (2018) *Nursing Practice: knowledge and care.* Chichester: John Wiley & Sons.

Pett, A. (2017) 'Getting the best out of others'. In Ashton, D., Ripman, J. and Williams, P. (eds) *How to be a Nurse or Midwife Leader.* Chichester: John Wiley & Sons.

Pollard, K. (2009) Student engagement in interprofessional working in practice placement settings. *Journal of Clinical Nursing,* **18(20):** 2846–56.

Quinney, A. and Hafford-Letchfield, T. (2012) *Interprofessional Social Work: effective collaborative approaches.* London: Learning Matters.

Royal College of Nursing (2018a) *Education: exploring roles within the education arm of nursing.* Available at: www.rcn.org.uk/professional-development/your-career/nurse/career-crossroads/career-ideas-and-inspiration/education (accessed 10 April 2019)

Royal College of Nursing (2018b) *RCN Credentialing: ALNP credentialing.* Available at: www.rcn.org.uk/professional-development/professional-services/credentialing (accessed 10 May 2019)

Thomas, J., Pollard, K. and Sellman, D. (eds) (2014) *Interprofessional Working in Health and Social Care: professional perspectives*, 2nd edition. Basingstoke: Palgrave Macmillan.

UK Government (2015) *Delivering Better Integrated Care*. Available at: www.gov.uk/guidance/enabling-integrated-care-in-the-nhs (accessed 10 April 2019)

Whittington, C. (2003) 'Collaboration and partnership in context'. In Weinstein, J., Whittington, C. and Leiba, T. (eds) *Collaboration in Social Work Practice*. London: Jessica Kingsley.

Useful websites

www.bnf.org (accessed 10 April 2019)
www.gov.uk (accessed 10 April 2019)
www.gov.uk/government/organisations/department-of-health-and-social-care (accessed 10 April 2019)
www.healthcareers.nhs.uk (accessed 10 April 2019)

REFLECTION AND CLINICAL SUPERVISION

This chapter looks at reflection as a learning strategy and the way in which it informs two specific aspects of professional development: clinical supervision and portfolios.

LEARNING OUTCOMES

On completion of this chapter you should be able to:
- understand the concept of reflection as a learning strategy
- describe the process of reflection and exercise the skills required to carry this out
- discuss the advantages of using reflection in practice
- appreciate how the reflective skills you develop as a student are carried on into registered nurse practice
- have an understanding of preceptorship
- appreciate the NMC's position on personal professional profiles
- consider how you might structure your own portfolio
- appreciate the concept and advantages of clinical supervision
- understand the need to build resilience

>> Reflection

Reflection is associated with learning from experience and is viewed as an important strategy for nurses, who should all embrace lifelong learning. The term 'reflection' is often used synonymously with the terms 'reflective practice' and 'reflective learning', and the literature about reflection indicates that most agree it is an active, conscious process where an experience is explored in order to gain new understandings and to learn something new.

- Dewey stated this as long ago as 1938 when he simply said: "we learn by doing and realising what we did" (Dewey, 1938, cited in Jasper *et al.*, 2013).
- Moon (2004) agrees with this when she states that reflective learning is where the learner considers their practice honestly and critically and is often initiated when the individual practitioner encounters some problematic aspect of practice and attempts to make sense of it.

- However, Jasper *et al.* (2013, p. 45) make the distinction between reflection and reflective practice: "using reflection alone in order to learn is not reflective practice... practice is about doing something. Therefore reflective practice means using the reflective process to inform practice in some way".
- Jasper *et al.* (2013) also point out that reflection is a learning strategy that can be achieved either formally or informally and can be outside the formal learning environment.

Reflection can help bridge the theory–practice gap that students often find so challenging: as a student you develop skills for learning in an educational setting (analysing literature, writing essays, etc.), whereas in practice you learn from the clinical setting, by working with your practice assessor and other healthcare professionals, performing new skills, assessing patients' needs, planning their care, etc. Reflection can help integrate these learning processes by using the theory gained from the educational setting to inform everyday working practices.

>> Reflection can help bridge the gap between theory and practice.

There are many different models for reflection, with no one being better than any other – it is a matter of personal choice which is used, but the consensus from nursing literature is that reflection should be structured to enable learning to result from it. Price (2002) suggests that reflection is more comfortable and effective if a step-by-step approach is used, and most of the reflective models acknowledge this, with a broad outline of the stages being:
- thinking back over a situation
- possibly discussing the incident with other people
- re-evaluating the experience to seek possible new understandings
- checking out new knowledge
- developing an action plan for the future.

(Mason-Whitehead and Mason, 2008)

Therefore good reflective practice underpins good professional practice, in that reflection enables practitioners to review their progress and identify areas which have been successfully developed, and those which are in need of further development. It enhances a commitment to 'lifelong learning' and continuous professional development.

>> Models of reflection

As mentioned above, there are many models of reflection to choose from. Outlined below are four of the most widely used:

Oelofsen's model

Oelofsen (2012) believes that reflective practice can be used to help nurses to make sense of work situations and, ultimately, to improve care. He proposed a simple, three-stage model, as shown in *Figure 9.1*.

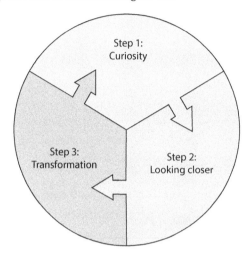

Figure 9.1: *The three-stage (CLT) model of reflection.*

Step 1: Curiosity. This step involves noticing things, asking questions and questioning assumptions. By doing this, nurses are trying to make sense of a situation and questions that help in this include:
- What exactly happened?
- Why did I/we deal with the situation in that way?
- What else could be happening?
- What was it like from the patient's perspective?
- What are my feelings about the situation?
- How did it affect me?
- What was the impact on us as a team when that happened?

Step 2: Looking closer. This step involves actively focusing on experiences and feelings about the situation being reflected upon, looking at the situation from a variety of perspectives and opening yourself to these perspectives, even if some of them may be contradictory. In this stage, reflective practitioners are challenging assumptions that underlie their own practice and that of others.

Step 3: Transformation. This phase is all about turning sense-making of a situation into action; by using observations from *Step 1* in conjunction with the insights gained from *Step 2*, the transformation phase is about finding ways to make positive change(s). The aim of change is to practise better and improve the care we give patients and significant others; this is called service improvement.

Gibbs' reflective cycle

Gibbs' (1988) reflective cycle (see *Figure 9.2*) is fairly straightforward and encourages a clear description of the situation, analysis of feelings, evaluation of the experience, analysis to make sense of the experience, conclusion where other options are considered, and reflection upon experience to examine what you would do if the situation arose again.

Stage 1: Description of the event

Describe in detail the event you are reflecting on. Include, for example, where were you; who else was there; why were you there; what were you doing; what were other people doing; the context of the event; what happened; what was your part in this; what parts did the other people play; what was the result?

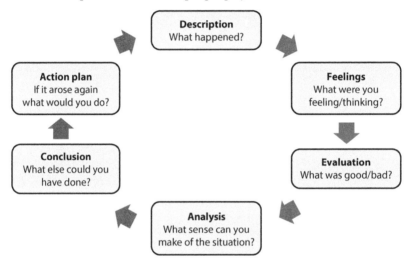

Figure 9.2: *Gibbs' (1988) reflective cycle.*

Stage 2: Feelings

At this stage try to recall and explore the things that were going on inside your head, i.e. why did this event stick in your mind? Include, for example: how were you feeling when the event started; what were you thinking about at the time; how did it make you feel; how did other people make you feel; how did you feel about the outcome of the event; what do you think about it now?

Stage 3: Evaluation

Try to evaluate or make a judgement about what has happened. Consider what was good about the experience and what didn't go so well or was bad about the experience.

Stage 4: Analysis

Break the event down into its component parts so they can be explored separately. You may need to ask more detailed questions about the answers to the last stage. Include, for example: what went well; what did you do well; what did others do well; what went wrong or did not turn out how it should have done; in what way did you or others contribute to this?

Stage 5: Conclusion

This differs from the evaluation stage in that you have now explored the issue from different angles and have a lot of information on which to base your judgement. It is here that you are likely to develop insight into your own and other people's behaviour in terms of how they contributed to the outcome of the event. Remember the purpose of reflection is to learn from an experience. Without detailed analysis and honest exploration that occurs during all the previous stages, it is unlikely that all aspects of the event will be taken into account and therefore valuable opportunities for learning can be missed. During this stage you should ask yourself what you could have done differently.

Stage 6: Action plan

During this stage you should think yourself forward into encountering the event again and plan what you would do – would you act differently or would you be likely to do the same?

Here the cycle is tentatively completed and suggests that, should the event occur again, it will be the focus of another reflective cycle.

Johns' (2010) model for structured reflection

Johns' (2010, cited in Bulman and Schutz, 2013) model for structured reflection can be used as a guide for analysis of a critical incident or general reflection on experience, and is useful for more complex analyses. Johns has refined his model over the years (he first wrote it in 1995) and he believes that the reflector should work with a supervisor, as he considers that through sharing reflections, greater understanding of those experiences can be achieved, rather than the reflector undertaking a lone exercise.

The stages of Johns' model of structured reflection are first to describe the experience and the significant factors, followed by reflection by asking:
- What was I trying to achieve? What are the consequences?
- What were the influencing factors? What things such as internal/external/ knowledge affected my decision-making?

- Could I have dealt with it better? What other choices did I have? What were the consequences of those?
- What have I learnt? What will change because of this experience? How did I feel about the experience?

From this learning you can reflect on how this experience has changed your ways of knowing. These are:

- empirics – scientific
- ethics – moral knowledge
- personal – self-awareness
- aesthetics – the art of what we do, our own experiences.

Rolfe, Freshwater and Jasper's framework for reflexive practice (2001/2011)

Whereas Gibbs (1988) and Johns (2006) proposed models for reflection, Rolfe *et al.* (2001) offer a framework for reflexive practice (see *Figure 9.3*). Although the words 'reflective' and 'reflexive' are often used interchangeably when referring to practice, there is a difference. Reflective models tend to focus on a retrospective analysis of a significant event or incident, without any real attempt to resolve the situation being reflected on.

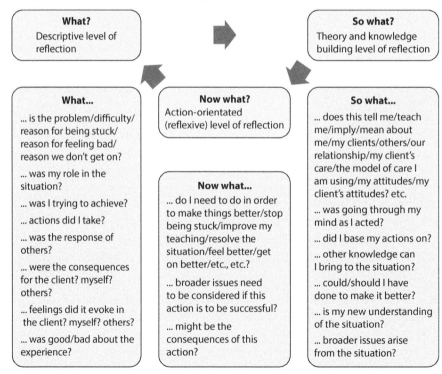

Figure 9.3: *Framework for reflexive practice (adapted from Rolfe et al., 2001).*

The Rolfe *et al.* model (2001) is based on Borton's framework (1970) which enables the practitioner to describe, make sense of and respond to a real-life situation by asking three questions – 'What?', 'So what?' and 'What next?'. However, where it differs from Borton's model is that the Rolfe *et al.* framework pays particular attention to the 'Now what?' action-orientated element, enables consideration of how the situation might be made better or changed in some way and encourages a plan of active intervention.

Driscoll (2006) has also used Borton's framework (1970) as the basis of a model for clinical supervision which is discussed later in this chapter.

>> Using reflective frameworks

Regardless of which model for reflection is used, Price (2002) suggests that the challenge of using reflective frameworks is often in ensuring that you have considered the following:

- Did you consider your own prejudices?
- Did you avoid seeing only the familiar and/or one perspective?
- Did you consider what others might have intended to signal through their behaviour?
- Did you make use of and check out all the available information?
- Did you actually learn something new?
- Did you form an action plan of how to approach this differently in future?

>> The benefits of practising reflectively

Jasper *et al.* (2013, p. 54) list the people and organisations they believe benefit from nurses practising reflectively. They are:

- the individual, in terms of providing individualised care, identifying their learning needs, and learning from experience
- the patient, in terms of higher quality and standards of care, and care designed to meet their own unique needs
- the employer, in terms of standards of care achieved, in having a continually developing workforce which recognises its own professional development
- the profession, in terms of self-regulation of the practitioners, in developing the nursing knowledge base, in contributing to increasing the status of nursing and recognition of nurses' contribution to patient care.

ACTIVITY 9.1

To see if Gibbs' reflective cycle can help you reflect on aspects of your practice, recall a recent clinical nursing situation in which you were involved. Write your description of the situation, and then apply the rest of Gibbs' model to reflect on the situation.

» Reflective writing – keeping a journal or reflective diary

The purpose of reflective writing is to support the process of reflection while, at the same time, providing evidence of learning (Oelofsen, 2012). It can take time to develop reflective skills, so it is important to build on this early in your course (Cottrell, 2019). Reflective writing requires a commitment of time and energy as it involves looking at a situation in depth, but it is an excellent basis for professional development, both as a student and when you become a registered nurse. The reasons that writing, rather than thinking or verbalising, is beneficial are that writing:

- is an active process
- organises and encourages deep thoughts and feelings
- enables the gaining of more control over thoughts, emotions, responses and behaviour
- encourages self-awareness, self-diagnosis and honesty
- encourages examination of the negative, development of the positive and can reveal uncertainties which need exploring
- is done for the purpose of learning
- provides a way of exploring a range of issues from different perspectives
- stimulates change.

(Jasper *et al.*, 2013; Cottrell, 2015)

Records of reflection over time should be kept in a portfolio as evidence of professional development and contribute to your personal development plan. This is essential for registered nurses, but it is also expected of students, and is good practice for them. It allows you to look for themes that recur and perhaps are not resolved, or conflicts that present themselves in a variety of forms. It also provides a safe base for you to explore your feelings; this can be challenging as you may discover truths about yourself which are embarrassing or make you feel uncomfortable. For this reason, Bulman and Schutz (2013, p. 215) suggest journals should be kept private and only selected aspects made available for more public reading.

Any of the frameworks already mentioned in this chapter can be used to write reflectively, or if you prefer you can write using 'free-flowing' text. As you become used to this process you will develop confidence in your own evaluation and judgement of your work. The important aspect is that you are writing about your experiences, so you should write in the first person. Focus on yourself, but avoid using reflection as a way of blaming or taking out anger on others; it is your own role you need to consider and how you would make a

> » Reflective writing involves writing about your own experiences, so you should write in the first person.

similar situation more manageable next time. Openness, honesty and critical analysis are the key features you need to consider, along with identification of any actions required in terms of your development.

Reflection is not all about 'clinical incidents'. You can reflect on your course by focusing on your development and progress as a whole, both academically and clinically. Cottrell (2019) suggests you consider:

- your feelings about your course, the lecturers, other students, your progress
- things you find difficult – challenges
- changes in your attitude or motivation
- how you tackle tasks – your strategies
- things you find out about yourself
- thoughts about how you learn best
- ideas that arise from your studies
- how different areas of studies link up
- how your studies relate to real life.

These aspects can act as a basis for discussion with your tutors, along with any possible options you may have to address any issues arising from your reflection.

RECAP

- Reflection can help bridge the gap between theory and practice.
- There are many models of reflection that have been developed and you can choose the one that suits you and the situation best.
- Reflective practice has benefits for you, for your patients and service users, for your eventual employer, and for the nursing profession as a whole.

ACTIVITY 9.2

Using a different model from that of Gibbs, write a short reflective account of a recent situation you encountered while studying at university (not a clinical event). Compare the reflective model used with Gibbs' model and consider which one you found the most useful.

» Preceptorship

There is a general acknowledgement that all professions need a period of transition following qualification for professional registration, and this of course includes nursing. The Department of Health (2010) published a Preceptorship Framework stating that all newly registered practitioners (nurses, midwives and allied health professionals) should undergo a period of preceptorship, defining this as:

"... a period of structured transition for the newly registered practitioner during which he or she will be supported by a preceptor, to develop their confidence as an autonomous professional, refine skills, values and behaviours and to continue on their journey of life-long learning"

(Department of Health, 2010, p. 11)

The precise length of preceptorship will vary according to individual need and local circumstances, but the Department of Health believes that six to twelve months is a suitable time. It acknowledges that every time a newly registered practitioner works alongside more experienced professional colleagues, they can learn from them and be guided by them in many ways. Formal preceptorship, however, means that the newly registered nurse is allocated a named individual, working in the same area of practice, who is on hand to guide, help, advise and support. The NMC states (2006, p. 1) that:

"... this doesn't mean that they accompany the newly registered nurse everywhere they go and constantly look over their shoulder, but it does mean they can be called if help is needed with a procedure or a situation not encountered before; or if they simply feel that they need support and guidance"

Preceptors, like practice supervisors and assessors, must be first-level registered nurses who have had at least twelve months' experience as a registered nurse and understand the concept of preceptorship. There are no formal qualifications to be a preceptor, but preceptors must (NMC, 2006, p. 1):

- know about the newly registered nurse's training and experience and be able to identify learning needs
- help the newly registered nurse apply knowledge to practice
- be able to act as a resource to facilitate the newly qualified nurse's professional development.

The content of a preceptorship programme is prescribed as including the following (Department of Health, 2010):

- team working
- decision-making
- confidence in applying evidence-based practice
- development of confidence and self-awareness
- implementation of codes of professional values
- increase of knowledge and clinical skills
- integrating prior learning into practice
- understanding policies and procedures

- reflection and receiving feedback
- development of an outcome-based approach to continuing professional development
- advocacy
- interpersonal skills
- management of risk and not being risk averse
- equality and diversity
- negotiation and conflict resolution
- leadership and management development.

Most NHS Trusts run preceptorship courses within their organisations. Some courses are affiliated to universities and nurses can gain academic credit for successfully completing the scheme of study.

Benefits of preceptorship are:
- enhanced patient care and experience
- improved recruitment and retention
- reduced sickness absence
- more confident and skilled nurses
- increased staff satisfaction and morale.

(NHS, 2018)

FURTHER READING

For more information about Preceptorships see:

Preceptorships for Newly Qualified Staff: www.nhsemployers.org/your-workforce/plan/education-and-training/preceptorships-for-newly-qualified-staff

An online preceptorship programme can be found at: www.flyingstart.scot.nhs.uk

---

>> Maintaining professional knowledge and competence (revalidation)

As previously stated, the Nursing and Midwifery Council exists to protect the public and it does this by making sure that only those who meet their requirements are allowed to practise as a registered nurse or midwife in the UK. Once you are a registered nurse you will have to go through the revalidation exercise every three years which:
- is the process that allows you to maintain your registration with the NMC
- builds on existing renewal requirements
- demonstrates your continued ability to practise safely and effectively, and
- is a continuous process that you will engage with throughout your career.

(NMC, 2016)

In order to renew your registration you must:

- have worked in some capacity by virtue of your nursing or midwifery qualification for a minimum of 450 hours during the previous three years (or have successfully undertaken an approved return to practice course within the last three years)
- undertake 35 hours of continuing professional development (CPD) (20 hours of which must be participatory) over the three years prior to the renewal of your registration
- obtain five pieces of practice-related feedback
- write five reflective accounts explaining what you learnt from your CPD activity
- record a reflective discussion with a registered nurse
- make a self-declaration of good health and good character
- provide evidence that you have professional indemnity cover
- have all the above confirmed by a 'confirmer'.

To help, the NMC provides lots of information about the revalidation process, at: http://revalidation.nmc.org.uk/welcome-to-revalidation/

» Continuing professional development and lifelong learning

Continuing professional development is defined as: "a process of lifelong learning for all individuals which meets the needs of patients and delivers health outcomes and health care priorities of the NHS which enables professionals to expand and fulfil their potential" (Department of Health, 1998, p. 194).

The study by Davis *et al.* (2014, p. 441) states that "lifelong learning in nursing is defined as a dynamic process, which encompasses both personal and professional life. This learning process is also both formal and informal. Lifelong learning involves seeking and appreciating new worlds or ideas in order to gain a new perspective as well as questioning one's environment, knowledge, skills and interactions. The most essential characteristics of a lifelong learner are reflection, questioning, enjoying learning, understanding the dynamic nature of knowledge, and engaging in learning by actively seeking learning opportunities. Keeping the mind active is essential to both lifelong learning and being able to translate knowledge into the capacity to deliver high quality nursing care". Therefore reflection and learning occur throughout your nursing journey and not just as a student nurse.

RECAP

- Preceptorship is a period of structured transition, usually between six and twelve months, to support newly qualified nurses to become confident and autonomous professionals.
- Maintaining your professional knowledge and competence and continuing your professional learning and development are important factors in the process of revalidation that all nurses undergo every three years.

» Clinical supervision

In *Chapter 1* we spoke about you having a practice supervisor and an assessor. When you are qualified you may have clinical supervision. This is a term that is used by registered nurses and other healthcare professionals to provide a purposeful, practice-focused relationship that enables the nurse to reflect on their practice with the support of a skilled supervisor (Peate, 2012). Clinical supervision was introduced in the workplace for nurses during the 1990s, following the Department of Health's document *Vision for the Future* (Department of Health, 1993) as a way of using reflective practice and shared experiences as part of continuing professional development (CPD). The concept, however, has long been established in professions such as midwifery, social work, psychotherapy and counselling.

Clinical supervision also has the support of the RCN (2003), which states that it enables registered nurses to:
- reflect on nursing practice
- identify solutions to problems
- increase understanding of professional issues
- improve standards of patient care
- further develop their skills and knowledge
- enhance understanding of their own practice
- identify room for improvement
- devise new ways of learning
- gain professional support.

Clinical supervision is different from any discussion you may have with your line manager when you are registered, in that it involves stepping back and reflecting on practice with a clinical supervisor who is external to your immediate workplace. It should not be confused with appraisal, development review or any other management activity. It is not currently a mandatory requirement from the NMC, and anything said in sessions should be confidential.

The clinical supervision sessions themselves should be carefully structured and managed with clearly defined aims and objectives. Ground rules and responsibilities should be clearly defined and there should be a contract of commitment from both supervisor and supervisees in order for it to be a meaningful exercise.

There are various models or approaches to clinical supervision; one-to-one supervision, group supervision, or peer group supervision. The choice of approach will depend on a number of factors, including personal choice, access to supervision, length of experience, qualifications, availability of supervisory groups, etc. However, everyone participating in clinical supervision will have a supervisor who is a skilled professional and assists other practitioners in the development of their skills, knowledge and professional values.

Fitzgerald (2000, p. 155) believes that:

> *"within these types of supervisory relationships reflection plays an important role in the clinical supervision process. The use of a reflective framework facilitates a structured approach to the agenda of the supervisory meeting and helps maintain the focus on practice whilst enabling a questioning approach."*

Driscoll (1994) suggested that not all reflective practice is clinical supervision, but all good supervision is potentially reflective practice. He also points out that clinical supervision is not only about reflecting on the big issues surrounding clinical practice, but also on the seemingly insignificant and most ordinary of practice activities.

>> Good clinical supervision can offer an opportunity for reflective practice.

Driscoll's (2006) model of clinical supervision is probably the most widely known and used. It is in the form of reflective practice, but the essential difference is that it involves another person helping someone to reflect. It is cyclical in nature and is known as the WHAT? It contains three elements, these elements being used for a supervisee to prepare for clinical supervision.

- WHAT? – a description of the event
- SO WHAT? – an analysis of the event
- NOW WHAT? – proposed actions following the event.

Driscoll (2006) also lists a number of trigger questions, which are not dissimilar to those posed by Johns (2010) and Stephenson (1994), but in addition he lists some skills and attributes required (of both supervisor and supervisee) for effective clinical supervision. They are:

- a willingness to learn from what happens in practice
- being open enough to share elements of practice with other people
- being motivated enough to replay aspects of clinical practice

- having knowledge for clinical practice, which can emerge from within, as well as outside clinical practice
- being aware of the conditions necessary for reflection to occur
- a belief that it is possible to change as a practitioner
- the ability to describe in detail before analysing practice problems
- recognising the consequences of reflection
- the ability to articulate what happens in practice
- a belief that there is no end point about learning in practice
- not being defensive about what other people notice about one's practice
- being courageous enough to act on reflection
- working out schemes to personally action what has been learned
- being honest in describing clinical practice to others.

» Resilience in nursing

Every healthcare provider has to face a number of stresses and difficult situations as they provide daily care for patients. This puts members of the healthcare profession at risk of anxiety, depression, stress-related illnesses and burnout. Nursing comes with plenty of unique stresses and high pressure situations and therefore resilience training and coping mechanisms are considered vital for managing a work–life balance. Resilience can be described as the ability to recover and recuperate quickly from a difficult or challenging situation. Resilience is also having the ability to understand that stress happens

> » Being a reflective practitioner and a lifelong learner will help you build resilience.

and is a normal part of work. A nurse who is resilient can give better patient care and patient outcomes because they are more alert and positive, practise clear communication and exercise good clinical judgement because they are motivated and can take on more responsibilities. Those who are resilient in nature will generally have:

- a higher sense of self-awareness
- persistence
- energy to sustain their mind and body
- emotional intelligence
- emotional flexibility
- adaptability
- a positive outlook
- the ability to reach out to others for open communication.

(Health Insights, 2017)

As healthcare is a complex, stressful and challenging profession you will need to build resilience to survive. Research suggests that reflective practice and seeking support when on practice placement are key to reaching qualification. Whilst reflective practice is integral to nurse education programmes, many have also incorporated resilience training and coping strategies.

FURTHER READING

Health Insights (2017) Resilience in Nursing. *HealthTimes*. Available at: https://
   healthtimes.com.au/hub/nursing-careers/6/practice/healthinsights/
   resilience-in-nursing/2353/

CHAPTER SUMMARY

- Reflection is an important learning strategy and encourages lifelong learning.
- Good reflective practice underpins good professional practice.
- There are many different models for reflection and no one is better than another.
- Reflection is personal but you may be asked to share your experiences with others.
- Once registered, you will be expected to keep a portfolio of your experiences (NMC, 2016).
- Resilience is a need to sustain nurse education and excellent nursing practice.

References

Borton, T. (1970) *Reach, Touch and Teach*. London: Hutchinson.

Bulman, C. and Schutz, S. (eds) (2013) *Reflective Practice in Nursing*, 5ᵗʰ edition. Chichester: John Wiley & Sons.

Cottrell, S. (2015) *Skills for Success: personal development and employability*, 3ʳᵈ edition. London: Palgrave Macmillan.

Cottrell, S. (2019) *The Study Skills Handbook*, 5ᵗʰ edition. London: Red Globe Press.

Davis, L., Taylor, H. and Reyes, H. (2014) Lifelong learning in nursing: a Delphi study. *Nurse Education Today*, 34(3): 441–5.

Department of Health (1993) *A Vision for the Future: the nursing, midwifery and health visiting contribution to health and health care*. London: HMSO.

Department of Health (1998) *A First Class Service: quality in the new NHS*. London: DH.

Department of Health (2010) *Preceptorship Framework for Newly Registered Nurses, Midwives and Allied Health Professionals*. London: DH.

Driscoll, J. (1994) Reflective practice for practice. *Senior Nurse*, 14(1): 47–50.

Driscoll, J. (2006) *Practising Clinical Supervision: a reflective approach for healthcare professionals*, 2ⁿᵈ edition. London: Baillière Tindall.

Fitzgerald, M. (2000) 'Clinical Supervision and Reflective Practice' in: Burns, S. and Bulman, C. (eds) *Reflective Practice in Nursing*, 2ⁿᵈ edition (Chapter 5). Oxford: Blackwell Scientific.

Gibbs, G. (1988) *Learning by Doing: a guide to teaching and learning methods*. Further Education Unit. Oxford: Oxford Polytechnic.

Health Insights (2017) Resilience in Nursing. *Health Times*. Available at: https://healthtimes.com.au/hub/nursing-careers/6/practice/healthinsights/resilience-in-nursing/2353/ (accessed 10 April 2019)

Jasper, M., Rosser, M. and Mooney, G. (eds) (2013) *Professional Development, Reflection and Decision-Making in Nursing and Healthcare*, 2nd edition. Oxford: Wiley-Blackwell.

Johns, C. (2006) *Engaging Reflection in Practice: a narrative approach*. Oxford: Blackwell Publishing.

Johns, C. (2010) *Guided Reflection*, 2nd edition. Oxford: Wiley-Blackwell.

Mason-Whitehead, E. and Mason, T. (2008) *Study Skills for Nurses*, 2nd edition. London: Sage.

Moon, J. (2004) *A Handbook of Reflective and Experiential Learning: theory and practice*. Abingdon: Routledge.

National Health Service (2018) *Preceptorships for Newly Qualified Staff*. Available at: www.nhsemployers.org/your-workforce/plan/workforce-supply/education-and-training/preceptorships-for-newly-qualified-staff (accessed 10 April 2019)

Nursing and Midwifery Council (2006) *Preceptorship Guidelines, 21/2006*. London: NMC.

Nursing and Midwifery Council (2016) *Revalidation*. London: NMC.

Oelofsen, N. (2012) *Developing Reflective Practice*. Banbury: Lantern Publishing Ltd.

Peate, I. (2012) *The Student's Guide to Becoming a Nurse*, 2nd edition. Chichester: Wiley-Blackwell.

Price, B. (2002) Effective learning No. 3: Reflective observations in practice. *Nursing Standard*, **17(9)**: S1–2.

Rolfe, G., Freshwater, D. and Jasper, M. (2001) *Critical Reflection for Nursing and the Helping Professions: a user's guide*. Basingstoke: Palgrave Macmillan.

Rolfe, G., Jasper, M. and Freshwater, D. (2011) *Critical Reflection in Practice: generating knowledge for care*. Basingstoke: Palgrave Macmillan.

Royal College of Nursing (2003) *Clinical Supervision in the Workplace:* Guidance for Occupational Health Nurses. London: RCN.

Stephenson, S. (1994) 'Reflection – a Student Perspective' in: Palmer, A., Burns, S. and Bulman, C. (eds) *Reflective Practice in Nursing: the growth of the reflective practitioner*. London: Blackwell Scientific.

STUDY SKILLS

The aim of this chapter is to provide a brief overview of some of the key factors associated with study skills.

LEARNING OUTCOMES

On completion of this chapter you should be able to:
- identify, discuss and make use of some key study skills
- make use of some key skills for researching information online

» Study skills

The term 'study' relates to applying the mind to acquire knowledge. Most of us probably never really think about the skills required for studying – we just get on and do it. However, the more study skills and strategies you apply and practise, the more independent and confident you can become in any learning situation. It should also be remembered that no two people study in exactly the same way, so what works for one person may well not work for another. The following section offers some widely recognised skills that you might like to try, to see if they work for you.

» Reading

When you start a nursing course, you will have the same problem as every other student – how to get through the vast amount of reading you are required to do in order to complete the programme. There will not be enough time to read everything line by line so you will have to learn the skills that enable you to read efficiently and effectively within the time you have available. The following provides a brief overview of some of the main skills involved.

> » You will need to learn how to read efficiently and effectively within the time you have available.

Environment

Before we look at reading skills, think about the environment in which you are reading. It is most unlikely that you will be able to concentrate on reading and understanding if you are in an environment that is noisy and uncomfortable. Try to find a physical environment that is conducive for you to read in, for example by turning off the television or moving into a quiet room, or using a library. Other things you might consider include making sure the lighting is adequate, and that you are comfortably seated and working at a table if you are going to take notes. Work out what time of the day is best for you to study, and read at this time whenever possible. Try to avoid important reading if you are tired or if your eyes ache.

Styles or types of reading

Your style of reading should be chosen to suit the task. Styles or types of reading include the following:

Skimming

This is the technique you may use when you are going through a newspaper or magazine. The idea is that you read quickly to get the main points, and skip over the detail. It's also useful to skim when reading academic text, to:
- preview a passage before you read it in detail
- refresh your understanding of a passage after you have read it in detail
- decide if a book in the library or bookshop is right for you – to do this look at the title, author, synopsis (on back cover or front flap), contents page and date of publication, for an indication of its relevance to your needs.

Scanning

Having decided on the potential usefulness of a book from your skim, you need then to confirm that it will indeed be useful to you for your studies. This involves a more in-depth examination or scanning of a text for specific information relevant to your task or topic area. This can include scanning:
- the synopsis on the back cover of the book
- the introduction or preface of a book
- the first or last paragraphs of chapters
- the concluding chapter of a book.

Detailed reading

This is where you read sections and chapters in full, identifying and extracting the main points or examples from the text.

Critical reading

Critical reading requires you to evaluate the information and arguments in the text. You need to distinguish fact from opinion, and look at arguments given for and against the various issues. This is also where, having read appropriately more than one text on a similar topic, you begin to identify and compare and contrast any bias, objectivity and perspective that they may have. Using such comparisons when writing an essay can help you to produce a balanced and objective piece of work.

Reading skills

Active reading

When you are reading for your course, in order to help maintain your concentration and understanding, you will need to make sure you are as actively involved with the text as possible. Active reading can include a variety of techniques:

- **Underlining and highlighting** – pick out what you think are the most important parts of what you are reading. If you are a visual learner, you will find it helpful to use different colours to highlight different aspects of what you are reading. (Please only do this with your own copy of texts or on photocopies, not with books or journals borrowed from the library, or from fellow students or lecturers).
- **Note keywords** – record the main headings as you read. Use one or two keywords for each point. When you do not want to mark the text, keep a folder of notes you make whilst reading.

SQ3R method

One well-recognised model of active reading that incorporates some of these suggestions is the SQ3R method. The method was introduced by Francis P. Robinson in his 1946 book 'Effective Study' (now out of print). Robinson was an American education philosopher and stated that the SQ3R method involved five steps which should, if followed, help you to get the most out of your reading. The five steps are:

1. Survey
2. Question
3. Read
4. Recall/recite
5. Review
   - S = **Survey** – This first step helps you to focus on the author's topic and purpose (what are they trying to get across to the reader?) and on main

ideas in the text. Before reading, you need to survey the material. This can involve looking briefly at the title of the chapter, any bold headings or subheadings, any visual aids to points such as charts, maps and diagrams, and reading the chapter introduction and summary. Only a few minutes need be spent surveying the text to ease you into the reading.

– **Q = Question** – This step requires deliberate effort. The key here is to develop a questioning attitude as you read the chapter or text. This can be achieved by, for example, turning the title, headings and/or subheadings into questions (e.g. if the subheading is 'recording references' your question may be 'why do I need to record references?'). It can also include looking at any questions that might be posed by the author through set activities or at the end of the chapter. Writing the questions down keeps you alert and helps focus your concentration on what you need to learn from your reading.

– **R = Read** – For this step you need to read the material actively and try to answer any of the questions you have raised. Note down and answer questions in your own words, as this will enable you to understand and comprehend more fully the text you are reading. Look for the main ideas and important details, notice italicised or bold words, study any visual aids and make sure you understand their meaning and relevance to the text. Reduce your reading speed for difficult passages of text, and stop and re-read parts that are not clear.

– **R = Recite or recall** – Keep challenging yourself to make sure you have an understanding of what you are reading, by recitation and constant recall. After each section, stop and think back to your questions. See if you can answer them from memory. If not, take a look back at the text. Try to recall main headings, important issues and concepts in your own words and what graphs and charts indicate. Do this as often as you need, as it can help you learn and apply the knowledge to other areas.

– **R = Review** – The review is an assessment of what you have accomplished. When you have finished a chapter, article, etc., go back over the questions you posed during your reading. See if you can still answer them. If not, look back and refresh your memory; re-read if necessary. The review is a good time to go over any notes you have taken to help clarify points you may have missed or don't understand. It can also be useful to make flashcards for important points or for those questions that you found difficult to answer. The best time to review is when you have just finished studying.

(Lobdell, 2019)

FURTHER READING

More information about the SQ3R method can be found on websites such as www.uefap.com and www.studygs.net.

>> Taking notes

Note-taking is a skill that you will need to use many times as a student of nursing. Effective note-taking should have a purpose and be well organised, and can be a time-saving skill. By making notes you actively process and interpret ideas and information; this aids concentration and understanding and should enable you to learn more. Notes can also play an important part in planning assignments and projects by helping you identify the main points and organise your ideas into a logical order. When preparing for an exam, notes can provide a concise record of information for you to revise from. There is no one 'correct' way to take notes. Everyone tends to develop their own way of taking notes, and very different approaches can be equally effective.

The following are tips on how you might become an efficient and successful note-taker. These can apply equally to taking notes from a verbal presentation or from a written text.

Amount

The whole point of note-taking is to be able to summarise information in a different, shorter form to use later. Whichever strategy you use, it is important to realise you do not have to copy down everything you read or hear. If you do, note-taking will just become time-consuming, ineffective and a boring and passive way of learning.

Keywords and phrases

When making notes, listen or look out for keywords and phrases such as 'the most important factor is'. In your notes, keywords and phrases should trigger your memory or lead on to other ideas or explanations, so they must be easy to find when you are reviewing your notes at a later date. This may be achieved by:

- underlining important points once, very important points twice
- using CAPITAL LETTERS
- drawing boxes around the keywords
- putting an asterisk * next to the main idea
- going over the most important points with a highlighter pen
- using different coloured inks for different themes or approaches.

Symbols and abbreviations

When you take notes, particularly in a lecture, seminar, etc., or even on clinical placement, you will rarely have time to write in full sentences, or sometimes even full words. It is therefore useful to develop your own set of symbols and abbreviations. Some of the more common ones, which you will probably already be aware of, include:

e.g.	for example	>	greater than
i.e.	that is	∴	therefore
+	and/plus	a/c	account
=	equals	no.	number
NB	note well	ref.	reference
%	percentage	vs.	against/as opposed to
etc.	and so on	w/	with
<	less than	w/o	without

Remember though – do keep a copy of any of your own abbreviations in the front of your notes file so that you can refer to them at a later date.

Mind mapping (spray diagram/spider diagram)

Mind maps offer a non-linear and diagrammatical way to organise key ideas from your lectures, seminars and reading. They also have the potential to present a large amount of information on one page and act as a summary for more detailed notes.

In a mind map the main topic or argument is placed at the centre of the page (see *Figure 10.1*).

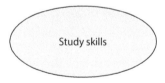

Figure 10.1: *Main topic of the mind map.*

Ideas that relate to the main topic are then placed on branches that directly connect to the central topic (see *Figure 10.2*).

Each of these main ideas then develops its own branches of ideas (see *Figure 10.3*).

As each theme is developed you add branch lines from each topic. Sometimes, it can also help to add colours and/or differently shaped boxes.

Once complete, and you have all your ideas down on paper, look for links between themes and indicate them with an arrow or chain. When using this technique for an assignment, exam, etc. it can be useful to number each theme to show the order in which you are going to refer to them.

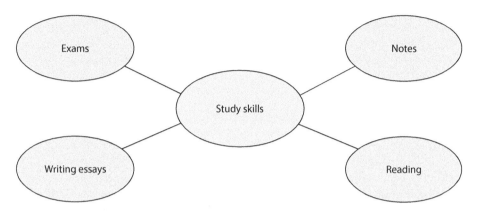

Figure 10.2: *Main branches of the mind map.*

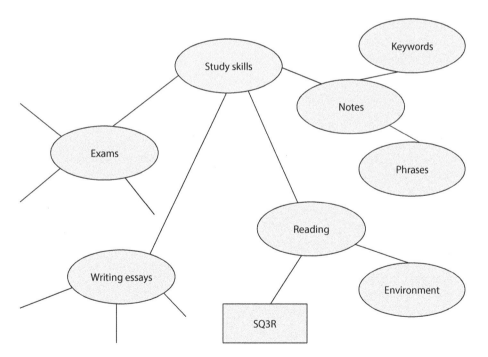

Figure 10.3: *Further branches.*

Handwriting, spelling and grammar

When you have completed a set of notes, check back and make sure that you can actually understand the notes you have made and that your handwriting has not become unreadable. Make any alterations while the topic is still fresh in your mind or when there are people present who can clarify what you should have written. As long as your meaning is clear don't worry about your spelling and grammar. At this stage it is better to focus on recording the information, so achieving perfection in spelling and grammar is not important – save this for your assignment or exam.

Plagiarism and paraphrasing in notes

Plagiarism can become an issue, especially when taking notes from written texts. In order to avoid this, do not just copy down material verbatim from another source without putting it in quotation marks and noting its origin – always put the full reference and page number in the margin beside the quote. If you do not do this, you may well forget that these words are not your own. If you then include them as your own in an assignment, report, etc., you will have committed plagiarism. It is better when taking notes to paraphrase (i.e. put a passage into your own words) wherever possible. However, you will still need to acknowledge the initial source of your information in your essay, etc. If you do this at the note-taking stage, there can be no confusion later on. Plagiarism is discussed in more detail in relation to essay-writing later in this chapter.

Organise your notes

Although it seems to be common sense, it is surprising how many people do not organise effectively the notes they take during their course of study. It is important to have a good system for organising and storing your notes, as doing this well will save you a great deal of time when it comes to using them when preparing for an assignment or exam. Whatever system you decide to use or develop, it should suit your personal needs. The following are some suggestions as to how your notes may be organised effectively.

- Use a separate file for each subject area.
- Use file dividers to separate major topics.
- Arrange notes under headings or questions.
- Number and label pages so that you can re-file them easily.
- Use one lecture note book per subject.
- Always leave a margin down one side of the page for future notes, references, comments, etc.

For more information see the *Useful websites* section at the end of this chapter.

RECAP

- The SQ3R method can help you get the most out of your reading.
- Make sure the notes you take are legible and well organised so you can understand them and use them effectively.

>> Writing essays

Writing essays is something that you will have to do on a regular basis in order to demonstrate your understanding of a topic in a well-structured written format. There is, once again, no single correct way to approach essay writing; you need to find what approach suits you best. The following section offers some tips to support or develop your approach.

Understanding the question

The basis of any essay should always begin from an understanding of what you are trying to achieve. It is therefore important to make sure that you know exactly what is required of you before you begin to research or to draft your essay. If you have been given a specific question, you need to begin by 'unpicking' the information it contains. This can be done by carefully examining the words of the question, looking for: the **content words** that indicate the subject matter with which the essay should deal; **limiting words** that specify the particular aspect or aspects of the subject on which the essay should focus; and the **instruction words** which tell you how to approach the topic.

Essay questions usually contain one or more of the following keywords that indicate what you are being asked to do:
- **Account for:** give reasons for, explain how something came about, clarify
- **Analyse:** examine in detail, consider the various parts of the whole and describe the interrelationship between them
- **Assess:** decide the importance/value of something and give reasons
- **Comment on:** explain the importance of
- **Compare:** examine the objects in question with a view to demonstrating their similarities
- **Contrast:** examine the objects in question for the purpose of demonstrating differences, or examine two or more opposing ideas or arguments to highlight their differences
- **Define:** state precisely the meaning of something using examples – a simple statement is often not enough; it needs to be explored in detail

- **Discuss:** explain and give different views about something – this can include your own views as long as they are based on sound evidence (i.e. they are referenced)
- **Evaluate:** examine the evidence and decide the value of something; make a judgement about it, based on sound evidence
- **Examine:** look at very carefully
- **Explain:** make very clear why something is the way it is, or why it happens
- **Give an account of:** describe in detail how something happened
- **Illustrate:** make something very clear, using evidence and examples
- **Outline:** give a short description of the main points
- **Justify:** support a particular idea, using evidence, and show why particular conclusions were made – include counter-arguments
- **Show:** make clear; demonstrate evidence for
- **Summarise:** outline the main points briefly.

Essay planning

Once you have decided what is required, researched the topic and read through your notes, you should then make an essay plan. Time spent on essay planning is rarely time wasted as it provides an opportunity to identify the main themes, sections or areas and how all the various pieces of information fit together. An essay plan is also useful to take to a tutorial so that you can discuss with your tutor your ideas about completing the assignment. The plan should be written in a way that works for you personally, for example as a mind map, linear notes or a set of boxes, etc.

Structure of an essay

The structure of the essay is important because it demonstrates that you are able to order your thoughts in a systematic, logical way and provides a sense of direction through the essay. The accepted basic framework for any essay is:
- introduction
- main text/body
- conclusion.

The introduction

The purpose of the introduction should be to set the context and direction of the essay. It should therefore:
- be clear that it is an introduction
- if required, set the question topic against a wider background (set the context)
- identify and/or define any key terms

- briefly summarise the overall theme of the essay, indicating the main points to be made and, possibly, the order in which they are to be presented – that is, explain what the essay is going to do.

Main text/body

The main body of the text is where the main ideas or arguments are developed. Depending on the length of the essay, it will contain several sections, each divided into paragraphs. The paragraphs should be logically linked as you develop the themes or ideas. In the main body you should:
- present key points clearly
- present ideas or arguments backed up by evidence from your reading
- accurately cite quotations and references to other works
- label any diagrams, figures or tables correctly.

Conclusion

The conclusion should follow logically from, and be based on, what you have presented in the main body of your essay as it brings together the main ideas explored. This can be achieved by:
- briefly summarising the main ideas and arguments
- linking back to the title/topic, showing how you have answered the question or drawn a relevant conclusion
- making clear why conclusions reached are important or significant
- not including any new ideas.

Referencing

Referencing is the standardised method of acknowledging sources of information. When writing an essay, report or dissertation, it is usual to make reference (i.e. to identify the place where the original citation can be found) to the sources that you have used, referred to, or taken quotes from. These references might be from, for example, journals, newspaper articles, books or book chapters, government reports or internet publications. When you refer to someone else's work or directly quote from it, you must acknowledge all the contributors and refer to all the authors/editors, both in the text and in a reference list or bibliography at the end of your work. Citing accurate references in academic work is important for the following reasons:
- to give credit to other authors' concepts and ideas
- to provide evidence of the extent of your reading
- to allow a reader to locate the cited references easily
- to avoid being accused of plagiarism (see below).

There are many systems for the citation of references, and you should follow the system that will be identified in your course handbook or assessment guidelines. The most commonly used systems in the UK are the Harvard system and the Vancouver system.

Harvard system

The Harvard system cites the author's surname and year of publication in the text, e.g. (Jones, 2004), and provides a reference list of any text citations in alphabetical order by author at the end of the assignment. It is here that additional details are noted, such as surname and initials, the title of the article, book or chapter, place of publication and the publisher.

Vancouver system

In the Vancouver system, a number is assigned to each reference as it is used. Even if the author is named in the text, a number must still be used. The original number assigned to the reference is used each time that reference is cited in the text. The first reference cited will be numbered 1 in the text, and the second reference cited will be numbered 2, and so on. If a reference cited number 1 is used again later in the text, it should be cited using the number 1 again. References are listed in numerical order in a reference list/bibliography at the end of the essay.

Please ensure you adhere to your individual educational organisation's referencing guidance.

Plagiarism in essay-writing

Plagiarism can be defined as: "the action or practice of taking someone else's work, idea, etc. and passing it off as one's own" (Oxford English Dictionary, 2017). This is a potentially serious offence in an academic environment, but it can easily be avoided by acknowledging all sources of information including social media, and ensuring data protection regulations are

>> Acknowledging all sources of information and referencing them will help you to avoid plagiarism.

upheld, as explored in *Chapter 3*. Failure to do this could result in work being downgraded, unmarked or/and disciplinary action taken.

Each university has strict guidelines on plagiarism. However, a basic guide is that the reference list should contain details of all the sources you have mentioned in your essay; a bibliography contains sources you have consulted but not mentioned in your essay. You may be asked for just a reference list or you may be asked for both references and a bibliography. You need to check your assignment guidelines to see what is required.

'Buying essays'

There are now multiple essay sites ('essay mills') where you can either purchase an essay or pay someone to write it for you. Some still suggest that their essay writing service is not cheating, that it is a good idea and that you will not be caught. **That is not true**; universities have complex software that aids detection, and buying essays is classified as plagiarism. Many universities take a high level of disciplinary action when a case of buying essays is detected because they do not want a cheat either in the university or in the caring/health profession when honesty and integrity are key parts of being a registered nurse and are in the *Code* (NMC, 2018).

A few final points about essays

Style of writing

Precision of language is very important. Ensure that your writing style:
- uses complete, straightforward sentences that are varied, not too simple or too convoluted (complex sentences do not necessarily signify complex thought), and also avoids writing in note form
- avoids using slang and colloquialisms
- only quotes relevant material and does not overuse quotes (it is much better to interpret information in your own words)
- does not use inappropriate analogies
- does not adopt a subjective or emotive tone
- does not make assertions or sweeping statements without supporting evidence or argument
- is not repetitive.

Paragraphs

There should be one main theme per paragraph and you should use paragraphs to signal the natural breaks in your argument when the focus of attention shifts. Excessively long paragraphs should be avoided and, where possible, the first sentence of each paragraph should link in some way to the previous paragraph. This allows for the flow or continuity of argument which is a very important quality in essays.

Link words

Link words are words that provide 'signposts' along the way, which help identify connections and relationships between key ideas. They include:
- words that lead the reader forwards, such as 'again', 'furthermore' and 'finally'
- words that make the reader stop and compare, such as 'however', 'although' and 'nonetheless'

- words that develop and summarise, such as 'clearly', 'therefore' and 'in conclusion'.

Length

The length of any assignment will be identified in the assignment guidelines. It is important that you are as close to your word limit as possible, as most universities or colleges will probably have clearly identified mark penalties if the word count of an assignment is more than 10 per cent over or under the stated amount for that piece of work. Usually it will be requested that you record your word count at the end of the assignment, and again failure to do so might result in the loss of some marks.

Proofread

The final preparation of the essay for submission is important. This includes carefully proofreading your essay, or asking a friend or relative to do this for you. Even better is getting someone to read your work back to you. Notice any faults of grammar and make sure you correct them before submitting the work. Spelling errors can sometimes be more difficult to detect, simply because you may not know how a particular word is spelt. Nevertheless, you should try to correct as many spelling errors as possible. Most word-processing packages include both spelling and grammar checks – use both but don't rely on them completely as some words may be spelt correctly but used in the wrong context such as, for example, 'there' and 'their'.

Electronic submission of essays

Almost all UK universities ask you to submit an electronic copy of your essay and a very few now ask for hard copies; however, the principles are the same as above regarding proofreading and ensuring your work is read for the marker. However, submitting your essay electronically has an added bonus because this is normally done via plagiarism detection software such as *Turnitin*. This software also allows you to submit your essay to test if you have inadvertently plagiarised, and if you use this test element of the software in a timely manner it will give you time to amend your work before you formally submit it by the appropriate deadline. The library services in universities will provide information regarding how to submit work electronically.

RECAP

- Make sure that you understand the question and plan your essay before you begin.

>> Electronic learning (e-learning)

E-learning is a unifying term used to describe the learning and delivery of a training or education programme using a computer or electronic device (for example, a mobile phone).

Some other terms frequently used interchangeably with 'e-learning' include:
- online learning
- online education
- distance education
- distance learning
- technology-based training
- web-based training
- computer-based training (generally thought of as learning from a CD-ROM).

Types of e-learning

E-learning comes in many variations and is often a combination of the following:
- purely online – no face-to-face meetings
- blended learning – combination of online and face-to-face
- synchronous – live interaction between tutor and students; students log in at a specific time and for a specified duration
- asynchronous – students learn through internet-based, network-based or stored disk-based modules; interaction with others includes via email, online discussion groups and online bulletin boards
- teacher-led group
- self-study
- web-based study
- computer-based (CD-ROM) study.

Features and benefits of e-learning

Wherever you look in the literature it is clear that the use of e-learning can demonstrate significant benefits. These benefits are that:
- learning is self-paced and provides the learner with a chance to speed up or slow down as necessary
- learning is self-directed, thus allowing a learner to choose content and tools appropriate to their differing interests, needs and skill levels
- range and course availability can be significantly increased
- it allows for multiple learning styles using a variety of delivery methods geared to different learners
- it tends to be more learner-centred
- accessibility is any time and anywhere

- online learning does not require physical attendance at a particular place and time
- it can encourage greater student interaction and collaboration
- it can encourage greater student/teacher contact
- it enhances computer and internet skills
- it provides global opportunities for learning.

(www.tech-faq.com; www.kineo.com)

>> Researching online

Some general tips include the following:

Narrow your research topic

The internet allows access to so much information that you can easily be overwhelmed. Before you start your search, think about what you're looking for and, if possible, formulate some very specific questions to direct and limit your search. Try not to use broad or general terms – rather, use terms that are more specific to the topic you are researching. You can also sometimes narrow your search by looking at sites that you may have previously used and that are relevant to your topic.

Boolean operators

Boolean operators are words that allow you to combine search terms and can be utilised in most search engines. The three most common are 'and', 'or' and 'not'.

- **and** – narrows the search and retrieves sites/records containing all the words it separates. For example, entering values AND ethics would instruct the search engine to find web pages that contain both words, 'values' and 'ethics'.
- **or** – broadens the search and retrieves sites/records containing any of the words it separates. For example, entering values OR ethics would cause the search engine to look for web pages that contain either the word 'values' or the word 'ethics', but not necessarily both words. You need to be mindful that this could result in the return of thousands or even millions of sites. 'Or' is most useful when the same term may appear in two different ways; such as, for example, typing evidence-based practice OR EBP to find information about evidence-based practice.
- **not** – narrows the search and retrieves sites that do not contain the term following the 'not' – i.e. it finds the first word but not the second. This limitation is helpful when you know your search term is likely to appear with another term that does not interest you, for example toddler NOT baby.

Exact phrases

If you want your search engine to search for an exact phrase, put double quotation marks around the phrase.

When searching you also need to include appropriate, alternative or synonymous terms. Scan the titles and abstracts of the sites/records you find for other possible keywords or synonyms you may not have thought of using. For example, a search on the common name 'St John's wort' finds records which include the Latin name *Hypericum* and the extract name 'hypericin'. A good revised search strategy would be: St John's wort OR hypericum OR hypericin.

Know your search engines and subject directories

Search engines (e.g. Google, Yahoo! and Bing) can differ considerably in how they work, how much of the internet they search, and the kind of results you can expect to get from them. Spending some time learning what each search engine will do and how best to use it can help you avoid a lot of frustration and wasted time later. There are a great many good academic resources available on the internet, including hundreds of online journals and sites set up by universities and scholarly or nursing organisations. The following are some bibliographic e-resources.

- The BNI (British Nursing Index) provides reference to journals and articles, some conference papers and major reports on aspects of education and nursing from the UK and some English language international publications.
- CINAHL (Cumulative Index to Nursing and Allied Health Literature) has international coverage and indexes nearly 5500 nursing and allied health journals.
- CRD (Centre for Reviews and Dissemination) enables the search of the Database of Abstracts of Reviews of Effects (DARE), the NHS Economic Evaluation Database (NHSEED) and the Health Technology Assessment database (HTA).
- The Cochrane Library is designed to provide evidence to inform healthcare decision-making.
- MEDLINE (Medical Literature Analysis and Retrieval System Online), ASSIA (Applied Social Science Index and Abstracts), IBSS (International Bibliography of the Social Sciences).

Evaluate the information

If you are not using recognised academic resources such as those above, you need to remember that anyone can put whatever they want on a website; there is no review or screening process, and there are no agreed standard ways of identifying subjects and creating cross-references. Therefore you must always think critically about the information you have found on the internet. Some of the questions you should be asking yourself are:

- Who is the author?
- Who is sponsoring the website?
- What is the audience level?
- Is the information current and up to date?
- Is the content reliable and accurate?

Remember that if you decide to use the information, you are responsible for ensuring that it is reliable and accurate.

(See also *Chapter 7* on 'Evidence-based practice' for hints on how to review articles.)

Keep a detailed record of sites you visit and the sites you use

Doing research on the internet inevitably means visiting some sites that are useful and many that are not. Keeping a record of useful websites is good practice so that you can revisit them at a later date. Also, if you are using the information in an essay or an assignment you can acknowledge the source of that information easily and accurately. Using the browser's history function for this is not really good practice as it will retain the web addresses or URLs of all the sites you visit, good or bad. In addition, if you are using a computer at your place of study, the memory in the history file may be erased at the end of your session. It is much better either to note down accurately on paper the sites you've found useful, bookmark them, or put onto a removable device such as a memory stick so that you will have a permanent record.

Double-check all URLs that you put in your paper

It is easy to make mistakes with complicated internet addresses, and typing errors will invalidate your references. If you type them into the location box of your browser you will be able to check that you have the correct address because it will take you to the site.

RECAP

- E-learning has benefits, such as being accessible any time and anywhere.
- It is important to think critically about information you find on the internet and to evaluate it carefully.

» Numeracy

Nurses adhere to 'seven rights' of medication administration: right medication, right client, right dose, right time, right route, right reason and right documentation; and part of this is correct calculation of the medication. During your nurse education you will have numerous amounts of teaching and practice regarding the eight routes of drug administration:

- Oral
- Sublingual and buccal routes
- Rectal
- Vaginal
- Topical
- Parenteral: intravenous (into a vein), subcutaneous (under the skin), and intramuscular (into muscle)
- Nasal
- Ocular/optic.

You will also have multiple chances to learn how to calculate medications safely, because the ability to perform drug calculations accurately is an essential skill for practising nurses in all settings around the world. Incorrect drug dosage in patients can result in under-dosing, overdosing leading to adverse side-effects, and at worst, death. Consequently the NMC requires all student nurses to pass drug calculation tests during and at the end of their course.

FURTHER READING

There is a considerable amount of information on the internet about study skills. You should be able to start your search using a general search engine such as Google.

The following books are highly recommended for anyone with a serious interest in long-term development of their learning and study skills:

Cottrell, S. (2019) *The Study Skills Handbook*, 5th edition. London: Red Globe Press.

Ghisoni, M. and Murphy, P. (2019) *Study Skills for Nursing, Health and Social Care*. Banbury: Lantern Publishing Ltd.

Means, B., Bakia, M. and Murphy, R. (2014) *Learning Online: what research tells us about whether, when and how*. London: Routledge.

Osmond, A. (2015) *Academic Writing and Grammar for Students (SAGE Study Skills Series)*. London: SAGE.

Redman, P. and Maples, W. (2017) *Good Essay Writing*, 5th edition. London: SAGE.

CHAPTER SUMMARY

- The more study skills and strategies you apply and practise, the more independent and confident you can become in a learning situation.
- The style of reading should be chosen to suit the task, i.e. skimming, scanning, detailed or critical reading, and should be as active as possible.
- To be effective, note-taking should have a purpose and be well organised.
- The basis of any essay should always begin from an understanding of what you are trying to achieve.
- The accepted basic framework for any essay is an introduction, a main text/body and a conclusion.
- Maths and drug calculations are essential for safe nursing care.

Further information

If you are nervous about numeracy and clinical calculations, start practising now.
There are many online sources or books that can help you, such as:
https://www.mathsisfun.com/numbers/long-division-animation.html
'Understanding numeracy questions for nurses' video: https://www.youtube.com/watch?v=sBuo5qKXgnQ
Davison, N. (2014) *Numeracy and Clinical Calculations for Nurses.* Banbury: Lantern Publishing Ltd.

References

Davison, N. (2014) *Numeracy and Clinical Calculations for Nurses.* Banbury: Lantern Publishing Ltd.

Lobdell, M. (2019) *Study Less, Study Smart. A guide to effective techniques and enhanced learning.* Createspace Independent Publishing Platform.

Means, B., Bakia, M. and Murphy, R. (2014) *Learning Online: what research tells us about whether, when and how.* London: Routledge.

Nursing and Midwifery Council (2018) *The Code: professional standards of practice and behaviour for nurses, midwives and nursing associates.* London: NMC.

Osmond, A. (2015) *Academic Writing and Grammar for Students (SAGE Study Skills Series).* London: SAGE.

Oxford English Dictionary (2017) Available at: https://en.oxforddictionaries.com (accessed 10 April 2019)

Useful websites

Academic skills: www.gre.ac.uk/studyskills/reading_skills (accessed 12 April 2019)
The benefits of e-learning: www.heartassociation.eu/5-reasons-why-e-learning-is-great-for-nurses-and-nursing-students/ (accessed 2 May 2019)
Mind maps:
- www.litemind.com/what-is-mind-mapping (accessed 12 April 2019)
- www.mindtools.com/pages/article/newISS_01.htm (accessed 12 April 2019)
Guides and tutorials: www.reading.ac.uk/library/study-advice/lib-sa-guides.aspx (accessed 12 April 2019)

PUBLIC HEALTH AND PROMOTING HEALTH AND WELLBEING

The aim of this chapter is to raise your awareness about public health and promoting health and wellbeing, which are an integral part of every nursing student's and registered nurse's roles.

LEARNING OUTCOMES

On completion of this chapter you should be able to:
- define public health and health promotion
- appreciate the contested nature of wellbeing
- identify the wider determinants of health and health inequalities
- explain public health priorities
- describe the importance of empowerment in order to change behaviour
- understand the nurse's role in promoting health

>> Why is public health and promoting health and wellbeing relevant to nursing?

"Failing to meet the fundamental human needs of autonomy, empowerment and human freedom is a potent cause of ill health."

(Marmot, 2006, p. 2081)

The NMC (2018a) standards state that "Registered nurses play a key role in improving and maintaining the mental, physical and behavioural health and well-being of people, families, communities and populations. They support and enable people at all stages of life and in all care settings to make informed choices about how to manage health challenges in order to maximise their quality of life and improve health outcomes. They are actively involved in the prevention of and protection against disease and ill health and engage in public health, community development and global health agendas, and in the reduction of health inequalities" (ibid., p. 10).

Within the wider context of health and social policy, all four countries of the UK seek to improve the public health of their populations (NHS Scotland, 2012; NHS England, 2014; Public Health Agency [NI], 2015 and Public Health Wales, 2015). This is increasingly important as there is a growing and ageing population with many people living with more than one long-term condition (co-morbidities). In addition, with the requirement for clinical and cost-effectiveness there is an emphasis on being, and remaining, healthy as well as reducing health inequalities. Notwithstanding the political, epidemiological and demographic factors that impact on health, it is the responsibility of all registered nurses to promote the health and wellbeing of the patients/clients with whom they come into contact. This is embedded not only in the NMC *Code* (2018b) but also, as we have seen, in the NMC standards (2018a) which require the registered nurse to have "the underpinning knowledge and skills required for their role in health promotion and protection and prevention of ill health" (ibid., p. 11).

>> It is the responsibility of all registered nurses to promote the health and wellbeing of their patients.

Nurses are well placed to promote health and use a range of public health interventions, as they are at the forefront of delivering face-to-face person-centred care in a variety of acute and community settings. The RCN's (2016) survey '*The Value and Contribution of Nursing to Public Health in the UK*' endorses this by stating that "nurses have the skills and are best placed to provide meaningful public health interventions across all health and social care settings as part of holistic patient-centred care" (ibid., p. 28) and that "nursing staff are an integral and fundamental part of the public health workforce" (ibid., p. 29).

This chapter will define public health, health promotion and wellbeing. It will provide an overview of the context of public health, outline the public health priorities, and summarise the wider determinants of health and health inequalities. Following on from this there is a discussion of the term 'wellbeing'. The chapter will conclude with consideration of health promotion, including a discussion on individual and community empowerment.

>> The context of public health

Definition

Wanless (2004) provided what is now an accepted definition. Public health is:

> "the science and art of preventing disease, prolonging life and promoting health, through organised efforts and informed choices of society, organisations, public and private, communities and individuals."

This definition makes it explicit that public health is everybody's business and that it is an overarching term that includes many differing health promotion approaches and interventions at individual, family and community levels.

Historical context

The roots of public health can be traced back to Edwin Chadwick (1800–90), a social reformer who sought to have the English Poor Laws of 1601 and 1834 amended and who reported on *The Sanitary Conditions of the Labouring Population* in 1842. He believed science could improve health.

Other studies followed, such as Charles Booth's *Life and Labour of the Working Class in England* in 1903, documenting poverty in London, and Seebohm Rowntree's *Poverty: a study of town life*, which explored poverty in York. Both studies highlighted the inequalities within society and established a link between poverty and poor health. Indeed, Rowntree developed the first measurement for poverty (Moreno-Leguizamon and Spigner, 2009). The work of John Snow (1854), mapping outbreaks of cholera and tracing the disease back to one water pump, contributed to the understanding of how disease was spread and his work was the beginning of modern epidemiology. Legislation has also played an important role in improving the health of the UK, with the first parliamentary Public Health Acts in 1848. The first Sanitary Act of 1866 made local authorities responsible for sewers, water and clearing streets, and developments such as Joseph Bazalgette's sewerage system for London contributed to reducing the spread of diseases such as cholera.

During the Second World War, William Beveridge's Report on *Social Insurance and Allied Services* was published (Parliament UK, 2019). Within this report he set out his vision to eradicate what he saw as the 'five evils' – want, disease, idleness, ignorance and squalor – by the development of the welfare state as we know it today. From this, the NHS (1948) emerged to provide free healthcare to all from the 'cradle to the grave' with a focus on eliminating disease. The Town and Country Planning Act (1947) led to slum housing being cleared and new homes being built and the Education Act (1944) ensured all children had free education until they were aged 15.

All of these social changes also contributed to improving the health of the UK's population and are now seen as the wider, or social, determinants of health. More recently, developments in genetics, as well as improved medicines and treatments of diseases, together with further parliamentary Acts, such as the Health Act (2006) which banned smoking in public places, have all contributed to an overall improvement in the health of the UK's population and to our understanding of what public health is today.

Public health priorities

Each of the four nations of the UK has a public health organisation to oversee their health and wellbeing and reduce health inequalities. These organisations are Public Health England, Public Health Scotland, Public Health Wales and the Public Health Agency in Northern Ireland. Each nation has its own strategy and priorities.

An overarching approach to public health practice is defined by the UK's Faculty of Public Health (FPH) which states that it:
• is population based
• emphasises collective responsibility for health, its protection and disease prevention
• recognises the key role of the state, linked to a concern for the underlying socio-economic and wider determinants of health, as well as disease
• emphasises partnerships with all those who contribute to the health of the population.

(FPH, 2016a)

According to the FPH (2016a), there are three overarching public health domains:
1. Health Improvement
2. Health Protection
3. Healthcare Public Health.

Improving the health of the population has a focus on individuals' health behaviours, together with individual risk factors associated with poor health outcomes. These include the wider determinants of health (see below) as well as the principal preventative factors to ill health, mortality and morbidity. The NMC (2018a) recognises that a registered nurse should identify and use all appropriate opportunities, making reasonable adjustments when required, to discuss preventative factors. These are "the impact of smoking, substance and alcohol use, sexual behaviours, diet and exercise on mental, physical and behavioural health and wellbeing, in the context of people's individual circumstances" (ibid., p. 11). Therefore discussions may focus on key public health priorities:
• smoking cessation
• reducing obesity
• healthy eating
• reducing alcohol consumption
• improving mental health (including patients with dementia)
• tackling solvent abuse
• promoting physical activity
• improving sexual health.

Protecting individuals' health includes the provision of the UK immunisation and vaccination programmes, which have reduced the number of deaths and morbidities from diseases such as measles, rubella and polio and led to the elimination of what were common communicable diseases such as smallpox. Vaccinations aim to provide immunity for diseases for the person they are administered to. However, those who have been vaccinated are less likely to infect others who have not been vaccinated for medical reasons or by parental choice. This is referred to as 'herd immunity' (Public Health England, 2013). For this to be achieved, 90–95% of the population needs to be vaccinated (Oxford Vaccines Group, 2016). Nurses are expected to have knowledge and understanding of "the principles of pathogenesis [the biology of a disease], immunology [the immune system] and the evidence-base for immunisation, vaccination and herd immunity" (NMC, 2018a, Clause 2.11).

» To achieve herd immunity, 90–95% of the population needs to be vaccinated.

Protecting health also includes assessing the health effects in relation to being exposed to environmental factors such as biological or chemical agents, radiation or polluted water (FPH, 2010). On a day-to-day basis, nurses protect health through "understanding and applying the principles of infection prevention and control" (NMC, 2018a, Clause 2.12).

Healthcare Public Health (HCPH) focuses on the strategic areas of planning, procuring and monitoring of healthcare services. The FPH (2016b, p. 1) defines HCPH as "concerned with maximising the population benefits of healthcare while meeting the needs of individuals and groups, by prioritising available resources, by preventing diseases and by improving health-related outcomes through design, access utilisation and evaluation of effective and efficient healthcare interventions and pathways of care". Therefore, implementing evidence-based practice, clinical effectiveness and clinical governance (see also *Chapter* 6) all contribute to this, as well as the use of evaluation and audit.

Global health issues

Globalisation is a contemporary issue which Walsh (2018, p. 78) states "refers to a range of processes that have the effect of bringing dispersed populations into closer contact, creating a single, integrated community of interest or independent society". Orme *et al.* (2007, p. 205) put it more simply by stating that it is "the growing interdependence between different peoples, religions and countries". In addition, there is economic interdependency between countries and the ease of international travel which means that we live in a world where public health issues have the potential to impact worldwide, including the UK population.

These issues include, but are not limited to, communicable diseases such as Ebola, tuberculosis and SARS; environmental factors such as diseases from mosquito bites, including Zika virus and malaria; natural disasters (e.g. flooding) and industrial disasters (e.g. nuclear accidents). The WHO (2007) report entitled *The World Health Report 2007 – A Safer Future: global public health security in the 21ˢᵗ century* identifies the need for global health security and for individual countries to work together to identify risks to health and seek ways to address these within the International Health Regulations of 2005.

» Determinants of health and health inequalities

For nurses to deliver holistic person-centred care or family-centred care, it is essential to be aware that our patients/clients/families are more than their diagnosis. They live within families and communities and there are many wider 'social' factors that impact on health. These are known as the social determinants of health which can impact on health outcomes (such as life expectancy) and diseases (such as lung diseases which can be caused by living in damp housing). Overall, the health of the nation continues to improve in the UK thanks to improved medical and healthcare and social conditions.

However, these improvements mask a widening gap between the health outcomes of the wealthiest and the most deprived people and communities. This is known as health inequality. Consequently, to improve these inequalities the NHS cannot work alone to prevent disease, as there are many other contributing factors that are local, national and international.

These wider determinants of health are presented in Dahlgren and Whitehead's (1991) model which places individuals and their unique factors that influence their health at the centre (e.g. age, sex and genes). This is then encompassed in several layers, as in a rainbow, of other factors that determine health which includes lifestyle (alcohol, obesity, smoking), social and community networks, living and working conditions and the socio-economic, cultural and environmental factors (see *Figure 11.1* and https://esrc.ac.uk/about-us/50-years-of-esrc/50-achievements/the-dahlgren-whitehead-rainbow/).

The reality of health inequalities means that "a boy born in one of the most advantaged 20% of neighbourhoods in 2015 can now expect to outlive his counterpart, born in one of the least advantaged 20% of neighbourhoods, by 8.4 years. In 2001, that gap was 7.2 years. For girls, the difference has risen from 5 years to 5.8 years over the same period" (Longevity Science Panel, 2018). This is because those in poverty have poorer living standards;

> » People living in poverty have poorer standards of living, poorer health and shorter life expectancy.

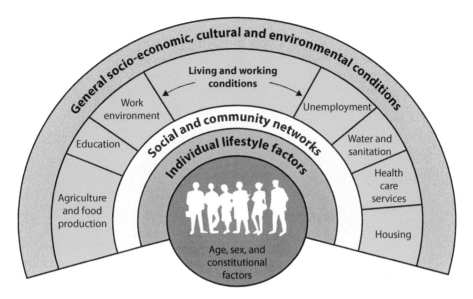

Figure 11.1: *The Dahlgren–Whitehead rainbow. Reproduced with permission from Institute for Futures Studies.*

for example, inadequate housing and diet. The Marmot Review (2010) highlighted a social gradient in health, where the less affluent a person's position, the worse their health. This review also described the importance of measures to address the wider determinants of health as well as interventions to prevent ill health by improving health behaviours, thereby reducing health inequalities and promoting health.

As identified, childhood has an influence on longevity and physical and mental health and wellbeing, as well as potential life choices. For example, studies such as those of Thacher *et al.* (2018) explore the relationship between parental smoking and asthma. Children living in poverty are more likely to "die in the first year of life, be born small, be bottle fed, breathe second-hand smoke, become overweight, suffer from asthma, have tooth decay, perform poorly at school [and] die in an accident" (Wickham *et al.*, 2016, p. 760).

Poverty, a wider determinant of health, is defined as having an income that is 60% of the median income in a year, measured after household costs are removed (McGuinness, 2018). There are an estimated 3.7 million children living in poverty (28% of children), almost one in three in the UK in 2013–14, despite 67% of these children having a parent in work (End Child Poverty, 2018). This can lead to poorer health outcomes and reduced educational attainment which in turn impacts on the choice and range of employment opportunities and less job security (Naidoo and Wills, 2016). Hence, health promotion interventions and public health initiatives are needed at individual, family and community levels.

FURTHER READING

Health inequalities have been well documented since the *Report of the Working Group on Inequalities in Health* (the Black Report) of 1980 which was assessed by Townsend and Davidson (1990) and in *The Health Divide* in 1987 (Whitehead, 1990). Further reports include those by Acheson (1988), Wanless (2004) and Marmot (2010) (focusing on England).

>> Local public health: Joint Strategic Needs Assessments (JSNA)

The Local Government and Public Involvement in Health Act of 2007 has required localities to produce a Joint Strategic Needs Assessment (JSNA) which seeks to inform the commissioning of health and social services, as well as the development of appropriate and effective services (Department of Communities and Local Government, 2005). This involves both statutory and non-statutory organisations such as the Local Authority (including Public Health which now sits within Local Authorities), local NHS organisations, service users, community and non-governmental organisations (voluntary sector) all working together to assess the local population needs and plan the current and future health and social care requirements in order to reduce health inequalities and improve health outcomes.

Therefore, this is a significant document when planning public health interventions and health promotion activities as it is important to address what the real need in a locality is, rather than the need a nurse or other practitioner thinks needs to be met; for example, an area with a high number of older people may have different priorities than an area with a high number of children. As such, the JSNA is a *top-down* approach to improving health; that is to say, the power for change and decision-making comes from these organisations.

RECAP

- Public health is the science and art of preventing disease, prolonging life and promoting health.
- Nurses have a responsibility to promote the health and wellbeing of their patients and to have the underpinning knowledge and skills required for this role.
- Factors such as lifestyle, social and community networks, living and working conditions and socio-economic, cultural and environmental conditions are all determinants of health.

ACTIVITY 11.1

Find the JSNA for your local area online. What are the needs identified and how are these needs being met? How can you as a nurse contribute to this?

>> Wellbeing

Today, the term wellbeing is part of our everyday vocabulary and is often linked with health and sometimes used synonymously. However, the WHO (1948) definition of health, "a complete physical, mental and social wellbeing and not merely the absence of disease", suggests wellbeing is an aspect of health. Hence wellbeing "incorporates subjective (self-perceived) feelings of happiness and contentment with spiritual and socio-economic factors" (Knight and McNaught, 2011, p. 1) and there is no commonly agreed definition.

The Department for Environment, Food and Rural Affairs (DEFRA) began measuring wellbeing in 2005 and the Office for National Statistics provides data on national and personal wellbeing. Subjective wellbeing can be researched using measurements of how happy people, or societies, feel and is often seen within psychological literature in terms of quality of life. However, this suggests that the quality of our lives is only determined by ourselves. As we have already noted, many factors impact adversely on health, and similarly on wellbeing.

McNaught (2011) sought to provide a definitional framework which illustrates the micro and the macro elements associated with wellbeing. Furthermore, he presents visually the notion that wellbeing is wider than the individual and encompasses family, community and society as a whole (see *Figure 11.2*).

It can be seen, using this definitional framework, that there is interlinking between an individual and their place within their family, their community (e.g. geographical or religious community) and society (job, influence of social policies, e.g. housing) as a whole. So the influences on wellbeing can be seen as multifactorial. Thus, individual wellbeing needs to be seen within this wider context as each individual's circumstances are unique to them. This is an important consideration for nurses when undertaking health promotion and forms the basis for person-centred approaches.

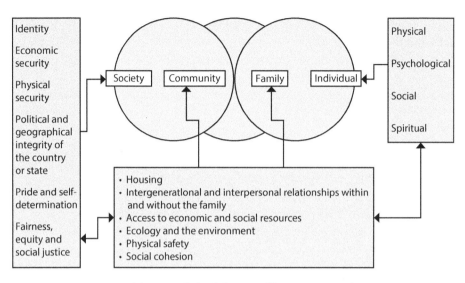

Figure 11.2: *A structured framework for defining wellbeing (McNaught, 2011, p. 11).*

>> Health promotion

The Ottawa Charter (WHO, 1986) states that:

> *"Health promotion is the process of enabling people to increase control over, and to improve, their health. To reach a state of complete physical, mental and social well-being, an individual or group must be able to identify and to realize aspirations, to satisfy needs, and to change or cope with the environment. Health is, therefore, seen as a resource for everyday life, not the objective of living. Health is a positive concept emphasizing social and personal resources, as well as physical capacities. Therefore, health promotion is not just the responsibility of the health sector, but goes beyond healthy life-styles to well-being."*

The WHO definition of health promotion is an important one as it acknowledges that individuals need to be healthy in order to live their daily lives; for example, participate in communities, families, work and so on. It recognises the wider determinants that impact on health, as discussed earlier in this chapter, and also makes it clear that the empowerment of individuals and communities is fundamental to health. Subsequently the WHO (2005) has reiterated this by stating that "Health promotion is the process of enabling people to increase control over, and to improve, their health. It moves beyond a focus on individual behaviour towards a wide range of social and environmental interventions." Health education, the giving of information and behaviour change, is one element of health promotion.

>> Empowerment and health education are fundamental to health promotion.

Within the NMC *Future Nurse* standards (2018a), Platform 2 (pp. 11–12) focuses solely on promoting health and preventing ill health (see also *Chapter 1*). The outcomes for this Platform aim to ensure that, at the point of registration, the newly registered nurse will have the underpinning knowledge and skills to undertake their role in health promotion and the protection and prevention of ill health. This is also embedded in the NMC *Code* (2018b) which specifies that nurses must:

"2.2.   recognise and respect the contribution that people can make to their own health and wellbeing

2.3.   encourage and empower people to share decisions about their treatment and care

3.1.   pay special attention to promoting wellbeing, preventing ill health and meeting the changing health and care needs of people during all life stages

3.3.   act in partnership with those receiving care, helping them to access relevant health and social care, information and support when they need it."

(NMC, 2018b, pp. 6–7)

There are many models for promoting health and these are not explored within this chapter. Nevertheless, whatever model is used, as both the WHO definitions and the NMC (2018b) make clear, empowerment of the individual or community is vital. Empowerment can be defined as "the act of acquiring power and the ability to make decisions and take control over one's life" (Naidoo and Wills, 2016, p. 75) and is a *bottom-up* approach to improving health.

This challenges the power relations between individuals and nurses: individuals have the freedom to choose and we, as nurses, cannot force them to make what we perceive to be a healthy lifestyle choice, even when based on the best evidence; e.g. stopping smoking. What we can do is boost an individual's self-confidence to identify and achieve their own 'healthy goal' and this can be seen as an empowering or strength-based approach.

Empowering people enables them to gain the knowledge, skill sets and attitudes to gain control of their lives and adapt to the changing world and their life circumstances. This can be achieved by using facilitation skills to enable individuals to develop their own coping mechanisms and/or personal skills (The Training Tree, 2017). Within this context, it is important to consider health literacy; i.e. an individual's ability to find health information and services and to understand the information to make an informed decision about their health (NMC, 2018b). As a nurse, you need to present information in an accessible, person-centred way to enable understanding (NMC, 2018b).

There are three key concepts associated with empowerment:

Self-esteem: self-esteem can be defined as "people's evaluations of their own self-worth—that is, the extent to which they view themselves as good, competent, and decent" (Aronson *et al.*, 2001, p. 19; cited by Sciangula and Morry, 2009). Self-esteem is central to an individual's personality, motivation and attainment in life (Walsh, 2018).

Self-efficacy: self-efficacy is defined as "the extent to which people believe they are competent to confront the challenges in life" (Niven, 2006, p. 365). An individual needs to feel that they have the power within them to make changes and that they are worthy of making this change. Furthermore, they need the coping strategies and skills to make the necessary changes to their behaviour in order to improve their health.

Locus of control: an individual's belief about whether they have control over their lives and health indicates that they have an internal locus of control. In contrast, if they believe they are subject to fate and are powerless they have an external locus of control (Niven, 2006, pp. 364–5).

Individual empowerment

One example of a brief health promotion intervention that can empower individuals and help them change their behaviour is Making Every Contact Count (MECC). This can be used in any health or social organisation and is:

> *"... an approach to behaviour change that uses the millions of day-to-day interactions that organisations and people have with other people to support them in making positive changes to their physical and mental health and wellbeing. MECC enables the opportunistic delivery of consistent and concise healthy lifestyle information and enables individuals to engage in conversations about their health at scale across organisations and populations."*

(Public Health England *et al.*, 2016, p. 6)

The focus is on having a 'healthy conversation'. Although this is an initiative in England only, it is an intervention that is transferable across all four countries of the UK as it is evidence-based. The use of MECC seeks to reduce health inequalities, prevent illness and improve health in a supportive way by empowering individuals to make changes.

The MECC principles ensure that this is a person-centred approach which treats the individual with dignity and respect and values their experience. It acknowledges that an individual is "the expert on themselves. Only they know what really interests, motivates or is important to them" (The Training Tree, 2017, p. 5). It is a method for a brief intervention which may only be for 30 seconds to five minutes. Between 30 seconds and two minutes equates to MECC level 1 (Very Brief Intervention) which is sufficient time to provide support and encouragement for individuals, or highlight a specific health issue and/or signpost them to resources (Public Health England *et al.*, 2016). MECC level 2 is a Brief Intervention which is longer than two minutes and "involves oral discussion, negotiation or encouragement, with or without written or other support or follow-up. It may also involve a referral for further interventions, directing people to other options, or more intensive support" (Public Health England *et al.*, 2016, p. 15).

As nurses we are aware that the conditions that are the major causes of premature death in the UK are cancer, heart disease, stroke, respiratory disease and liver disease, and the lifestyle factors associated with these are smoking, alcohol, obesity and lack of activity (NHS Choices, 2018). Hence, the focus of nurses can be concentrated on, for example, smoking cessation, reducing alcohol intake, having a healthy well-balanced diet and reducing weight. However, what is important to the individual needs to be elicited and may include a physical, mental or emotional health and/or wellbeing goal.

Central to a successful MECC interaction are effective communication skills (see also *Chapter 2*). The essence of the structure used is "Ask, Advise, Assist in order to have a [healthy] conversation which is based on the person's needs, goals, concerns and strengths" (The Training Tree, 2017, p. 3). This requires the nurse to be confident, use open questions to elicit information, actively listen and reflect on what is being said. The nurse can assist in goal setting; for example, using the SMART framework as a guide (Specific, Measurable, Achievable, Relevant and Time-bound) and expanding it to be SMARTER by including an evaluation (E) and when the goal will be reviewed (R). The nurse also needs to have the knowledge and skills to signpost individuals to appropriate and local services and resources. Indeed, it can be argued that for nurses to work in an empowering way, they themselves need to feel empowered.

ACTIVITY 11.2

Reflect on an individual health promotion activity with a patient/service user that you have either undertaken or observed. What factors contributed to it being an empowering interaction and how could it be improved further?

Community empowerment

In contrast to individual empowerment, community empowerment is:

"a process by which communities gain more control over the decisions and resources that influence their lives, including the [social] determinants of health. Community empowerment builds from the individual to the group to the wider collective and embodies the intention to bring about social and political change".

(Laverack, 2007, p. 29)

The WHO (2017) identifies that for community empowerment to be achieved there needs to be collective participation. Nevertheless, the WHO makes it clear that a community may not be geographically linked, but could have shared issues or characteristics: for example, a virtual social media group with a shared interest such as politics, gardening or cooking. The strength of this is that collectively, the community can have a greater influence and control over their quality of life in their defined community (WHO, 2017).

An example of a geographical community project is the Cultivating Lives Project, Grow Your Own Club. This project aimed to improve community cohesion on the Isle of Sheppey (Mehmet and Stacey, 2014). The Isle of Sheppey is an area of high socio-economic deprivation and the Cultivating Lives project was initially begun by a volunteer and an independent charity "to support social and environmental regeneration through community engagement" (ibid., p. 89). It was developed by the South East Coastal Communities and funded by the Higher Education Funding Council and became a joint project with the community and two universities in order to grow food, plants, shrubs and trees locally within a community garden. The outcomes included not only access to fresh food and plants, but also social connection, thereby reducing isolation by encouraging individuals to work together (such as clearing the land) and increased community knowledge of horticulture and agriculture.

The UK Men's Sheds Association can also be seen in terms of community empowerment. This Association supports local opportunities for men to meet and practise practical skills and be creative (in sheds or somewhere similar). Currently there are 444 across the UK (UK Men's Sheds Association, 2018). They provide an opportunity for men to meet and converse with other men, which addresses the loneliness and isolation many men feel as they may have fewer social connections than women. Indeed, it is well documented that loneliness and isolation have an impact on health and wellbeing (Milligan *et al.*, 2015). Many Men's Sheds also participate in local community projects (UK Men's Sheds Association, 2018).

ACTIVITY 11.3

Read Platform 2 of the NMC document *Future Nurse: standards of proficiency for registered nurses*. In the area where you live or in which you are a nursing student, explore online what local community initiatives exist which aim to improve quality of life; for example, a community chef team, gardening club or community exercise group such as Walking for Health. Consider how you could contribute to and become actively involved in a community empowerment project such as these.

CHAPTER SUMMARY

- Nurses have an important role in public health and health promotion in relation to the health and wellbeing of individuals, families, communities and populations.
- Opportunities in clinical practice should be sought to discuss "the impact of smoking, substance and alcohol use, sexual behaviours, diet and exercise on mental, physical and behavioural health and wellbeing, in the context of people's individual circumstances" (NMC, 2018a).
- Empowering individuals, families and communities is an important aspect of changing behaviours.
- The wider determinants of health have an influence on an individual's life expectancy and health inequalities.
- Each of the four countries of the UK has a public health strategy, with local areas identifying their own specific health and social care needs.

Further information

- Knight, A., La Placa, V. and McNaught, A. (2014) *Wellbeing: policy and practice*. Banbury: Lantern Publishing Ltd.
- Knight, A. and McNaught, A. (2011) *Understanding Wellbeing: an introduction for students and practitioners of health and social care*. Banbury: Lantern Publishing Ltd.

References

Acheson, D. (1988) *Public Health in England: report to the committee of inquiry into the future of the public health function*. London: HMSO.

Dahlgren, G. and Whitehead, M. (1991) *Policies and Strategies to Promote Social Equity in Health*. Stockholm: Institute for Futures Studies.

Department of Communities and Local Government (2005) *Sustainable Communities: people, places and prosperity*. Cmnd 6425. London: HMSO.

End Child Poverty (2018) *Key Facts*. Available at www.endchildpoverty.org.uk/key-facts/ (accessed 12 April 2019)

Faculty of Public Health (2016a) *Good Public Health Practice Framework 2016*. Available at: www.fph.org.uk/media/1304/good-public-health-practice-framework_-2016_final.pdf (accessed 26 April 2019)

Faculty of Public Health (2016b) *Healthcare Public Health: ensuring sustainability and capability of Healthcare Public Health across the system*. Available at: www.sph.nhs.uk/wp-content/uploads/2016/03/Healthcare-public-health-capability-in-England-March-2016.pdf (accessed 26 April 2019)

Knight, A. and McNaught, A. (2011) 'Introduction'. In: Knight, A. and McNaught, A. (eds) *Understanding Wellbeing: an introduction for students and practitioners of health and social care*. Banbury: Lantern Publishing Ltd.

Laverack, G. (2007) *Health Promotion Practice: building empowered communities*. Maidenhead: Open University Press.

Longevity Science Panel (2018) *Widening Rich–Poor Mortality Gap* (press release). Available online at: www.longevitypanel.co.uk/_files/Press_release_2018.pdf (accessed 12 April 2019)

Marmot, M. (2006) Health in an unequal world. *Lancet*, **368**: 2081–94.

Marmot, M. (2010) *Fair Society, Healthy Lives*. London: The Marmot Review.

McGuinness, F. (2018) *Poverty in the UK: statistics*. House of Commons Briefing Paper Number 7096, 23 April 2018. London: House of Commons Library.

McNaught, A. (2011) 'Defining wellbeing'. In: Knight, A. and McNaught, A. (eds) *Understanding Wellbeing: an introduction for students and practitioners of health and social care*. Banbury: Lantern Publishing Ltd.

Mehmet, N. and Stacey C. (2014) 'Green space and wellbeing'. In Knight, A., La Placa, V. and McNaught, A. (eds) *Wellbeing: policy and practice*. Banbury: Lantern Publishing Ltd.

Milligan, C., Payne, S., Bingley, A. and Cockshott, Z. (2015) Place and wellbeing: shedding light on activity interventions for older men. *Ageing and Society*, **35(1)**: 124–49.

Moreno-Leguizamon, C. and Spigner, C. (2009) 'Theory, research and practice in public health'. In: Stewart, J. and Cornish, Y. *Professional Practice in Public Health*. Exeter: Reflect Press.

Naidoo, J. and Wills, J. (2016) *Foundations for Health Promotion*, 4ᵗʰ edition. Edinburgh: Elsevier.

NHS Choices (2018) *The Top Five Causes of Premature Death*. Available at: www.nhs.uk/Livewell/over60s/Pages/The-top-five-causes-of-premature-death.aspx (accessed 12 April 2019)

NHS England (2014) *The Forward View into Action: planning for 2015/6*. Leeds: NHS England.

NHS Scotland (2012) *A Route Map to the 2020 Vision for Health and Social Care*. Edinburgh: NHS Scotland.

Niven, N. (2006) *The Psychology of Nursing Care*. Basingstoke: Palgrave Macmillan.

Nursing and Midwifery Council (2018a) *Future Nurse: standards of proficiency for registered nurses*. London: NMC.

Nursing and Midwifery Council (2018b) *The Code: professional standards of practice and behaviour for nurses, midwives and nursing associates*. London: NMC.

Orme, J., Powell, J., Taylor, P. and Grey, M. (2007) *Public Health for the 21st Century: new perspectives on policy, participation and practice*, 2ⁿᵈ edition. Maidenhead: Open University Press.

Oxford Vaccines Group (2016) *Herd Immunity: how does it work?* Available at www.ovg.ox.ac.uk/news/herd-immunity-how-does-it-work (accessed 10 April 2019)

Parliament UK (2019) *Living Heritage. People and Parliament Transforming Society. 1942 Beveridge Report*. Available at: www.parliament.uk/about/living-heritage/transformingsociety/livinglearning/coll-9-health1/coll-9-health/ (accessed 25 April 2019)

Public Health Agency (2015) *Annual Business Plan 2015–2016*. Belfast: Public Health Agency.

Public Health England (2013) *The Green Book*. Available at www.gov.uk/government/collections/immunisation-against-infectious-disease-the-green-book (accessed 10 April 2019)

Public Health England, NHS England and Health Education England (2016) *Making Every Contact Count (MECC): Consensus statement*. London: Public Health England.

Public Health Wales (2015) *A Healthier, Happier and Fairer Wales: our strategic plan 2015–2018*. Cardiff: Public Health Wales.

Royal College of Nursing (2016) *The Value and Contribution of Nursing to Public Health in the UK: final report.* London: RCN.

Sciangula, A. and Morry, M. (2009) Self-esteem and perceived regard: how I see myself affects my relationship satisfaction. *Journal of Social Psychology,* **149(2)**: 143–58.

Thacher, J., Gehring, U., Gruzieva, O. *et al.* (2018) Maternal smoking during pregnancy and early childhood and development of asthma and rhinoconjunctivitis – a MeDALL project. *Environmental Health Perspectives,* **162(4)**: 1–13.

Townsend, P. and Davidson, M. (1992) 'The Black Report'. In: Townsend, P. and Davidson, N. (eds) *Inequalities in Health,* 2nd edition. London: Penguin.

The Training Tree (2017) *MECC Workbook.* Available at: www.makingeverycontactcount.co.uk/media/1041/013-mecc-workbook-db-health-pdf.pdf (accessed 12 April 2019)

UK Men's Sheds Association (2018) *What is a Men's Shed?* Available at: https://menssheds.org.uk/about/what-is-a-mens-shed/ (accessed 12 April 2019)

Walsh, M. (2018) *Key Topics in Social Sciences: an A–Z guide for student nurses.* Banbury: Lantern Publishing Ltd.

Wanless, D. (2004) *Securing Good Health for the Whole Population: final report.* London: DH.

Whitehead, M. (1992) 'The health divide'. In Townsend, P. and Davidson, N. (eds) *Inequalities in Health,* 2nd edition. London: Penguin.

WHO (1986) *The Ottawa Charter for Health Promotion.* Available at: www.who.int/healthpromotion/conferences/previous/ottawa/en/ (accessed 12 April 2019)

WHO (2005) *Health Promotion.* Available at www.who.int/topics/health_promotion/en/ (accessed 12 April 2019)

WHO (2007) *The World Health Report 2007 – A Safer Future: global public health security in the 21st century.* Available at: www.who.int/whr/2007/whr07_en.pdf (accessed 12 April 2019)

WHO (2017) *Community Empowerment.* Available at: www.who.int/healthpromotion/conferences/7gchp/track1/en (accessed 12 April 2019)

Wickham, S., Anwar, E., Barr, B. *et al.* (2016) Poverty and child health in the UK: using evidence for action. *Archives of Disease in Childhood,* **101(8)**: 759–66.

INDEX